D0526707

PLATE I

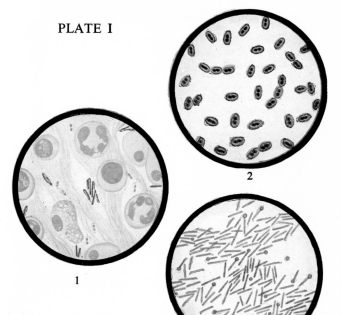

1. *Myco. tuberculosis* in sputum.

2. *Str. pneumoniae* stained to show capsules.

3. *Cl. tetani* stained to show spores.

4. *B. anthracis* stained to show spores.

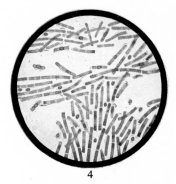

Nurses' Aids Series

MICROBIOLOGY FOR NURSES

NURSES' AIDS SERIES

ANATOMY AND PHYSIOLOGY FOR
NURSES
ARITHMETIC IN NURSING
EAR, NOSE AND THROAT NURSING
MEDICAL NURSING
MICROBIOLOGY FOR NURSES
OBSTETRIC AND GYNAECOLOGICAL
NURSING
ORTHOPAEDICS FOR NURSES
PAEDIATRIC NURSING
PERSONAL AND COMMUNITY HEALTH
PHARMACOLOGY FOR NURSES
PRACTICAL NURSING
PRACTICAL PROCEDURES
PSYCHIATRIC NURSING
PSYCHOLOGY FOR NURSES
SURGICAL NURSING
THEATRE TECHNIQUE
TROPICAL HYGIENE AND NURSING

NURSES' AIDS SERIES

Microbiology for Nurses

formerly Bacteriology for Nurses

E. JOAN BOCOCK

SRN, SCM, DN(London), RNT

Educator for Post Registration Studies, Victoria Hospital, Candos, Mauritius. Formerly Sister Tutor, St Thomas's Hospital, London, and Principal Tutor, Royal Free Hospital, London

With the assistance of
The Medical Staff of the Department of Microbiology
of the Royal Free Hospital, London

With Foreword by
NUALA CROWLEY

MRCS, LRCP, FC Path

Reader in Bacteriology, Royal Free Hospital

THIRD EDITION

LONDON
BAILLIÈRE, TINDALL & CASSELL

BACTERIOLOGY FOR NURSES

First Edition, January 1959
Reprinted October 1960
Reprinted September 1961
Second Edition, September 1962
Reprinted April 1965
Reprinted November 1966

MICROBIOLOGY FOR NURSES

Third Edition, August 1968
Reprinted November 1969

SBN 7020-0263-1

© 1968, Baillière, Tindall & Cassell Ltd.
7–8 Henrietta Street, London W.C.2

Published in the United States
by the Williams & Wilkins Company, Baltimore

Made and printed in Great Britain
by The Garden City Press Limited, Letchworth, Hertfordshire

FOREWORD

THIS book sets out to provide an introduction to the principles of bacteriology and immunity for nurses and to show how these apply to nursing procedures and the prevention of infection. Infectious diseases and cross-infections are always with us, though new patterns are slowly evolving through the influence of hygienic measures, antibiotics and immunization programmes. It is essential that nurses, whether senior or junior, should understand the principles involved in control of infection, which is hardly possible without knowing a little about the nature of bacteria and viruses. It has therefore been a pleasure to learn that this book has been very successful and filled a real need for nurses in training, without adding a heavy burden of specialized knowledge to an already crowded curriculum. I hope the new edition, which has been revised with particular reference to methods of sterilization, will be as successful as its predecessors.

NUALA CROWLEY

May, 1968

ACKNOWLEDGMENTS FOR ILLUSTRATIONS

I gratefully acknowledge permission to reproduce illustrations as follows: for Figs. 3, 4 and 5 the Director of the Wellcome Historical Museum, for Fig. 10 Vickers Instruments, for Fig. 35a Dr H. G. Pereira and the *Journal of Molecular Biology*, for 35b Dr Pereira and the *British Medical Bulletin*, for Figs. 36 and 37 Longmans, Green & Co. Ltd, for Figs. 38 and 39 the British Sterilizer Co. Ltd, and for Fig. 40 Laboratory Thermal Equipment Ltd. The colour plates and the micro-photographs of bacteria are taken from *Bacteriology and Immunology for Students of Medicine* by Stewart with permission of my present publishers, as also are Figs. 44–48 from *Theatre Technique*.

PREFACE

THE need for a suitable small textbook explaining microbiology to the student nurse and its relationship to the treatment and nursing care of the sick has been proved. I was glad and privileged to share in the preparation of the first two editions of this volume in the Nurses' Aids Series. I am delighted that a third edition has been called for, although I have greatly missed the help of Miss Armstrong my co-author in the first two editions, for her clear, logical mind and her mastery of the written word were invaluable.

In this third edition the text has again been most carefully revised and new material from the varied fields of microbiology has been added whenever it was required. In accordance with the widening scope of bacteriology departments this textbook, like them, has had its title altered to *Microbiology*.

How much microbiology the student nurse should be taught is a matter on which there can be divergent opinions, but if there should be any who think that the book goes more deeply into the subject than is necessary or desirable, I still say that it is better to err on the side of giving the nurse the opportunity of learning a little more, rather than a little less, of a subject which plays such an important part in her training and the care of the patient. Certain of the material, notably the tabular matter in the appendices, is of a kind which is suitable for reference rather than for memorizing, and as such it will be useful to the student nurse in connection with her everyday nursing experience. It is noteworthy that every disease mentioned in Chapter 8 has been seen at the

Royal Free Hospital during the last few years and that questions about each one of them have at various times been put to the Microbiology Department by nurses who were looking after those suffering from that disease.

I hope that both teacher and student will find helpful the suggestions in Appendix IV for the making of a glossary of difficult terms. The practical work suggested in the book, if carried out in schools of nursing, will prove a most valuable means of encouraging the intelligent management of the nursing techniques essential both for overcoming a primary infection for which the patient may be admitted or for preventing cross infection, which can seriously lengthen his stay in hospital.

I am again most grateful to Dr Nuala Crowley for her continuing interest in the book, and particularly for bringing the chapter on viruses up to date and for writing a foreword. I would also like to thank Dr Mark Ridley of the Department of Clinical Microbiology, St Thomas's Hospital, and Mr T. Hadgraft, Chief Pharmacist of the Royal Free Hospital, for their most valuable advice, and Mr R. H. Pyne, Head of the Central Sterile Supply Department of St Thomas's Hospital, who has given me much useful information on the new types of autoclave and the effects they have had on sterilizing techniques.

E. JOAN BOCOCK

April, 1968

CONTENTS

PLATES

ix

certainly remember lecturing to you, but I cannot see that you gained much benefit from the course', and he looked pointedly at the nurse's neck, round which dangled her discarded mask.

It may help those who, like this nurse, fail to appreciate the practical nature of bacterial and virus life, if they consider how differently the history of this country and of the world might have developed if the science of microbiology had earlier reached its present stage of fulfilment. The Prince Consort might not have died of typhoid fever in December 1861 and thousands of deaths from typhus might not have occurred in the First World War. In the Second World War things might have finished very differently if, by that time, penicillin and DDT had not been discovered.

Facts like these, tragic loss on the one hand and the wonders of prevention and cure on the other, may still be observed in any family or country. The determining factor today is the situation as regards the social services rather than, as in the past, lack of knowledge.

To nurses more than to most sections of the community are given both the knowledge and the opportunity of practising what has been learnt. This book has been written to further an earnest hope that the practice of nursing will be based in the future on an even more conscientious application of sound microbiological knowledge and principles. Since it has been written for student nurses it has been applied mainly to the hospital field. Nevertheless, the principles it embodies are of the greatest importance in the home, in the community and in every sphere of nursing experience.

2 BACTERIA AND OTHER MICROORGANISMS

Bacteria

BACTERIA are minute unicellular organisms ranging in size from $0.3\,\mu$ to $14\,\mu$ in length ($1\,\mu = \frac{1}{1000}$ mm). Ten of the smaller organisms could be placed end to end on the diameter of a red cell, and thirty red cells could fit across the diameter of a pin's head; bacteria cannot therefore be seen with the naked eye, and the high power or oil-immersion lens of a microscope is necessary to make out the shape of individual organisms. Each bacterium, however, is a functioning living unit, deriving its food from the surroundings in which it finds itself and using this food to manufacture the complex materials necessary for life and reproduction.

Bacteria vary enormously in the substance which they can utilize as food and there are some bacteria in nearly every situation where steps have not been taken to remove them; in the soil, in hot springs, in the sea, high in the air, in vegetable matter and on animals and in dust, their type depending upon the available foodstuff and the prevailing physical conditions. Some organisms are particular and require exacting conditions, perhaps the existence of animals or insects upon which they live, and the presence of the organisms will depend upon the presence of these animals or insects, which are said to act as vectors or carriers. The organism causing plague is found in rats; fleas bite the rats, become infected with the bacteria, and convey them to human beings. Ridding an area of rats therefore eliminates plague.

4

Not all bacteria, however, are harmful; indeed many are essential and a great many are useful. A large group of soil bacteria have the power of using atmospheric nitrogen for their growth; as they grow, reproduce and die, organic nitrogenous material is liberated into the soil enriching it and making it available to plants which have not this power of 'fixing nitrogen'. Bacteria in the soil elaborate vitamins necessary for animal life, and bacteria in the healthy bowel synthesize vitamins essential to human well-being. Bacteria are used to turn curd or cream into cheese, and the products of yet other bacteria turn grape juice into wine and wine into vinegar. These reactions are side reactions, which cannot be carried out in a laboratory or can be carried out only very slowly.

The term bacteriology therefore covers the study of a vast number of organisms, by far the greater number of which are not met with in medical work and do not cause disease. Those which are encountered in medical bacteriology have, for generations of organisms and centuries of time, become accustomed to living on organic material or animal tissues, and many have lost the power of using simple inorganic substances as a source of food; they have become to a lesser or greater degree parasitic.

Bacteria are of differing shapes,* which can be easily observed when they have been suitably stained and are

* The names of different types of bacteria are derived from Greek and Latin words denoting shape or other characteristic, or, in some cases, from the name of the discoverer of the organism. *Bacterium* is derived from Greek, from the diminutive form of the word *baktron*, a rod. The word, however, has been loosely used for all microorganisms, whatever their shape. *Coccus* is derived from the Greek word *kokkos*, a berry. *Spirochaete* stems from two Greek words: *speiro*, a coil, and *chaite*, flowing hair. *Bacillus* derives from the Latin *baculus*, a rod. Because of the use of the term bacteria for all organisms, bacillus has been widely used for rod-shaped organisms. Although pathologists have returned to the use of bacterium and prefer it to bacillus, the latter term is still much employed in general medicine.

examined with a high-powered lens on an ordinary microscope (the oil-immersion lens, p. 40). Some varieties are surrounded by a soft jelly-like material, the capsule, which may have a thickness greater than the diameter of the bacteria which it surrounds. Bacteria may be either

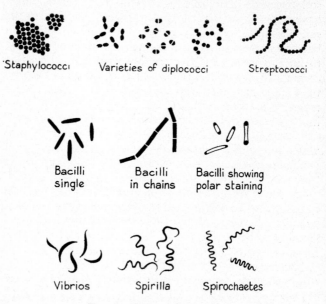

Staphylococci   Varieties of diplococci   Streptococci

Bacilli single   Bacilli in chains   Bacilli showing polar staining

Vibrios   Spirilla   Spirochaetes

FIG. 1.—TYPES OF BACTERIA.

round, when they are said to be coccoid and are often referred to as *cocci*; or rod-shaped, when they may be called *bacilli*. The term *vibrio* is used to describe a micro-organism which is rigid and has a single curve, e.g. the organism that causes cholera. Longer rigid, curved organisms usually with several spirals are termed *spirilla*, while *spirochaetes* are still longer, but flexible, spiral organisms.

The cocci are divided into several groups in accordance with the way in which they are arranged. They may be arranged in clusters, when they are termed *staphylococci*, or in pairs, when the term *diplococci* is applied to them, or in chains, when they are known as *streptococci*.

Bacteria do not contain a nucleus such as is to be seen in the larger cells which form either unicellular plant or animal organisms or the tissues of multicellular organisms such as man and the oak tree. Some bacteria are motile, that is, they are able to move of themselves, while others are merely carried about in moving currents of air or water, or in the dust and dirt particles that these may carry. Those that can move of themselves may do so because they possess a few or many little hair-like processes, called *flagella*, which have a lashing movement. This is the case with the bacilli which cause typhoid fever and can be seen when living specimens are examined under the microscope, or more easily by means of films made by a cine-camera through a microscope. Flagella are not found in the coccoid group of bacteria. Movement also occurs in the spirochaetal organisms by a bending of their spiral bodies, and the rate and character of the movement is characteristic. Again this can be seen under the microscope or by means of cine-films taken with suitable lighting or staining techniques. Some of the larger microorganisms which cause disease are of the *amoeba* class, and have the same amoeboid movement that is characteristic of those white blood cells which are able to pass out of the blood capillaries and engulf and devour bacteria when they get into the body tissues.

Bacteria require food and water like other living things. Lack of food and absence of water will cause their death. Some bacteria require oxygen and others will flourish only in its absence. Organisms which require oxygen are termed *aerobes*, and those which do not are called *anaerobes*. Bacteria which need oxygen will be found on the surface of wounds and on skin and mucous membranes, for example the organisms which cause sepsis in wounds and produce colds and other respiratory diseases. Bacteria which do not need oxygen and cannot grow in its presence will particularly affect deep wounds such as stab wounds and deep gunshot wounds; they include the

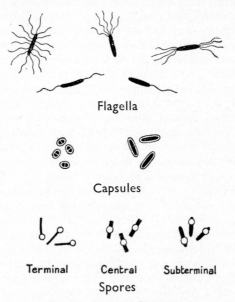

Flagella

Capsules

Terminal   Central   Subterminal
Spores

FIG. 2.—TYPES OF BACTERIA.

bacteria which cause tetanus and gas gangrene. Sometimes these infections may occur in open wounds because there is a mixed infection, and other bacteria present in the wound use up the oxygen available and so produce conditions in which anaerobic organisms can flourish.

Certain groups of organisms, notably those which cause anthrax and the *Clostridium* group responsible for tetanus and gas gangrene, have, in certain circumstances, the power of rounding off a part of their living material into compact balls; these balls are known as spores. Spores are extremely resistant to changes in temperature and to other killing agents and can survive in a state of suspended animation without moisture or food. They are like the seeds of plants which survive without food or water for months and even years, but grow and mature again when a suitable temperature and the food and water essential for life become available. The presence of spores may be demonstrated by special staining techniques.

Viruses and Rickettsiae

There is another group of infective agents, the viruses, which, like the bacteria, include pathogenic and non-pathogenic members and show an extreme degree of parasitism; they are dependent for life and reproduction on living cells which they invade; they make use of animal and plant, including even bacterial cells, some-times living a harmless mutual existence, when they are called commensals, and sometimes causing disease. The viruses differ from the bacteria in that they cannot be seen with an ordinary microscope, since they vary in size from 10 to 300 millimicrons (1 mμ = $\frac{1}{1000}$ μ), but they can be seen with an electron microscope.

A further group of organisms is the *rickettsiae*. Their characteristics appear to be midway between those of the bacteria and of the viruses. They vary in size from 300 mμ to 1000 mμ.

The presence of bacteria and other microorganisms therefore depends upon the availability of suitable food which the bacteria can take up and use, and upon the physical conditions, i.e. temperature, humidity, acidity and alkalinity, being favourable to their growth. Bacteria and viruses vary in the length of time during which they can stand adverse conditions and still remain alive. The organism causing tetanus can remain alive in the soil for many years, although the conditions are adverse for growth, by reason of its ability to form a protective coat or spore. It does not grow, but it does not die, while the gonococcus, the causative organism of gonorrhoea, will die in half an hour if it is allowed to dry in the air at room temperature.

3 THE HISTORY OF MICROBIOLOGY

THE history of microbiology is short but progress has been very rapid since the importance of bacteria as a cause of infectious disease has been recognized. Exact bacteriological diagnosis and to a large extent the diagnosis of virus disease is now possible. Epidemics can be controlled and preventive medicine can do much to limit disease, and some outbreaks, like diphtheria epidemics, have been practically eliminated. The advance in modern surgery has come about only since, as E. G. D. Murray says 'It has been lifted out of the despond of laudable pus into the security of asepsis'.

For centuries all races used the products of bacterial growth and fermentation, without realizing the implications of the changes or the processes involved. In fact the relationship between fermentation and infectious disease was not suspected until two centuries after bacteria were first seen in 1676, by Antonius van Leeuwenhoek, using primitive microscopes of his own design and making.

In 1546 Fracastoro wrote a book on contagion and was the first to record that infection is composed of minute insensible particles and proceeds from them. He noted that the infection was the same for 'he who received as for he who had given' the infection. This was a great advance, recognizing as it did the transmission of disease. Nevertheless, although contagion was generally recognized in some diseases, as in the plague and in syphilis, in others it was still missed.

11

In 1776 Spallanzani first cultivated bacteria in sterilized media, with and without air. He failed, however, to realize the importance of this and either was unaware of Fracastoro's work or failed to relate it to his own.

While this work was being carried on by the scientists, the cause of infectious disease was being investigated empirically by the clinicians of the day. In 1767 Hunter, investigating the causative organism of syphilis, experimentally infected himself. Unfortunately he induced in himself a mixed infection of gonorrhoea and syphilis and his results were, because of this, confused. In 1796 Jenner introduced vaccination, making use of the practical belief that those who had cowpox were immune or partially immune to smallpox.

It was not until 1847 that Semmelweis used the principle of ordinary social cleanliness to prevent sepsis. Dirt on instruments and skin acts as a binding agent for organisms, so the removal of extraneous dirt and grease did much to cut down sepsis by the removal of many of the pathogenic organisms and was a great step towards aseptic techniques.

The improvement in the microscope led to special diseases being associated with certain organisms of characteristic morphology. Davaine in 1850 saw what he called minute 'infusoria' in the blood of sheep dead from anthrax and he was able to transmit the disease by inoculation of greatly diluted blood. Subsequent work by Pasteur and Koch proved to be the starting point of microbiology.

The techniques of modern microbiology have developed greatly since the science was begun by pure chemists, headed by Pasteur whose interest began with industrial fermentation problems. He demonstrated that alcoholic fermentation was brought about by specific bacterial enzymes, and gave a logical explanation for a process which had been carried on for hundreds of years. Pasteur's studies were widespread, involving the ripening and preserving of wine, diseases of silkworms, and putrefaction.

Lister followed Pasteur's work on fermentation and carried out experiments to test the deduction that if

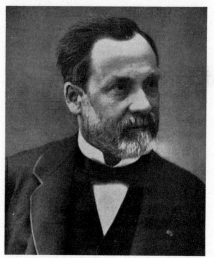

(*Wellcome Historical Medical Museum*)

Fig. 3.—Louis Pasteur (1822–1885).

fermentation of sugar and starch was due to bacterial action, sepsis and putrefaction of proteins were due to a similar cause. He therefore attempted to prevent bacterial infection of operation wounds and injuries and the many forms of sepsis which resulted in suppuration, hospital gangrene and septicaemia. He used carbolic, or phenol, to destroy germs and prevent them gaining access to wounds, and published the successful results of his work in *The Lancet* in 1867, though it was a long time before many of his sceptical colleagues accepted his teaching. By applying carbolic putty to cases of compound fracture, he was able to save limbs which would previously have been amputated because of the risks of a fatal result from gangrene or septicaemia. He made it

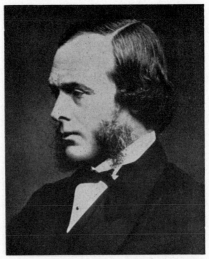

(*Wellcome Historical Medical Museum*)

FIG. 4.—LORD LISTER (1827–1912).

possible to operate safely within the abdominal cavity and on joints and bones, developments which later, with further advances in asepsis, antisepsis and anaesthetics, made every part of the body accessible to surgery.

While Pasteur was working in France and Lister in England, Koch in Germany was developing bacteriological techniques which form the basis of modern diagnostic bacteriology. Today it is relatively simple to identify an unknown organism. The tests which are likely to be of use under given conditions have now been laid down (the routine in chemical analysis to discover an organism might be likened to police work to discover a wrongdoer), but in 1870 Koch had no such rules to help him and new disciplines had to be worked out. Koch

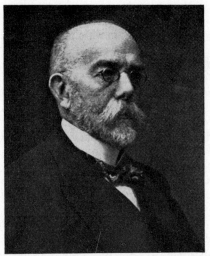

(*Wellcome Historical Medical Museum*)

FIG. 5.—ROBERT KOCH (1843–1910).

isolated the bacillus of anthrax, and this was the first pathogenic organism to be isolated in culture free from other organisms. He devised liquid and solid culture media which include both serum and blood agar and noted that the organism grew in clusters called colonies which eventually became visible to the naked eye. He saw that these colonies were characteristic and had defined conditions of growth. After this start the causative organisms of numerous other infectious diseases were isolated and their conditions of growth noted in the same way.

In 1881 Klebs and Loeffler isolated the diphtheria bacillus and later workers grew tetanus organisms. The discovery of these organisms necessitated a reassessment of the preformed theories of bacterial infection. It was discovered that filtrates of growing cultures of these organisms, that is to say material in which the organisms had been growing but from which they had been removed by means of filtration, were still able to cause death from diphtheria. This led to the discovery of toxins, or powerful tissue-poisons, often enzymes or ferments, which are produced by some organisms during growth and secreted into the surrounding tissues to be carried through the body in the blood stream. Organisms like the bacilli causing diphtheria and tetanus were found to be capable of growing in one part of the body and producing poisons which could be transmitted widely by the tissue fluids, blood or nerves.

In 1890 von Behring showed that diphtheria could be prevented and cured by the administration of serum from a horse recovered from diphtheria. This was the discovery of antitoxins. In 1891 Ehrlich standardized diphtheria toxin so that its potency could be assessed and the antitoxin measured against it.

Metchnikoff, studying inflammation in 1883, called the polymorphonuclear white cells present in pus 'phagocytes' and he put forward the theory that these cells were protective in that they destroyed and engulfed the infecting bacteria.

Less is known about the viruses than about bacteria. As has already been stated they are too small to be seen by the ordinary microscope although they can now be seen with the electron microscope. They will not grow on artificial media but require living cells inside which they multiply, that is to say they are intracellular parasites and their metabolism is closely bound up with the metabolism of the host cell. For these reasons the classical methods of study used in bacteriology are inapplicable and new ones have been, and are being, devised.

4 INFECTION AND IMMUNITY

Infection

IN nature a host is one who gives house room and nurture. An organism which invades the tissues of a host, finds a suitable place to multiply, leaves this host and invades another, is said to be a *pathogenic organism* if during its passage through the host it does harm. This is an important definition because many organisms live on mucous membranes, on the skin and in the gut, but do not 'invade'. On the other hand, some invade through the mucous membranes or skin, and even enter the blood stream on occasion, but do no damage and are quickly killed and removed by the body's defence mechanism. The route of transmission may be direct or indirect (Figs. 6, 7), and in either case infection may occur between two different hosts, i.e. cross-infection or between two sites on the same host, i.e. auto-infection.

The invading organisms can cause damage in one of three ways:

(*a*) They may invade and therefore destroy vital cells, e.g. in the way that the virus of poliomyelitis settles in the nerve cells.

(*b*) They may invade some mechanically important structure so that it is made inefficient, for example the organism of syphilis attacks the wall of the aorta, so that it is weakened and bursts. Old beams which are riddled with death watch beetle are weakened in a similar way.

(c) They may produce, while growing, a chemical poison which interferes with some essential process of the host; for example tetanus toxins affect nerve cells and diphtheria toxins damage both heart muscle and nervous tissues.

Thus to be an effective pathogenic agent an organism must be able to invade or get into a susceptible host; it can do no harm if it cannot get into the tissues even though it produces the most lethal of toxins in its growth. It must be able to find a suitable place to multiply before it is killed by the defences of the body. The tetanus bacillus is a normal inhabitant of the faeces and frequently gets into wounds. It comparatively rarely causes disease because its spores can germinate only under anaerobic conditions, that is where there is no oxygen. Where free air is available it cannot grow. In war wounds with much dirt and dead tissue the conditions become anaerobic or oxygen-free, the spores germinate, the organisms grow, and the disease of tetanus is produced.

The Spread of Infection. Having produced the disease in one host, a pathogenic race of organisms, if it is to continue, must be transmitted to another host or the race will die out. This attribute of communicability is a complex one depending upon many factors, of which only a few can be mentioned here.

Perhaps the most important factor in communicability of pathogenic organisms is the site of the lesion in the infected host or the place of maximum concentration of the organism. If this is in the throat, as for instance with a haemolytic streptococcus in a case of tonsillitis, this organism will be coughed or breathed into the surrounding air. The force with which it is expelled will determine how far from the infected host the organism will travel.

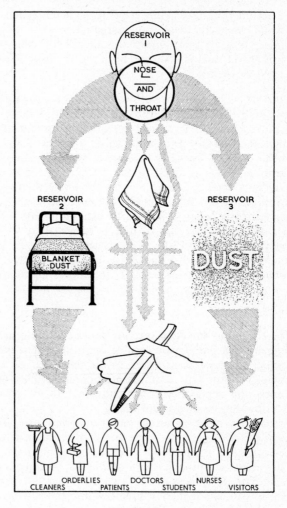

Fig. 6.
The Spread of Infection through Inhalation.

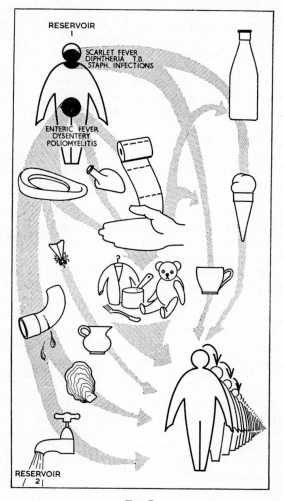

FIG. 7.

THE SPREAD OF INFECTION THROUGH INGESTION.

The same haemolytic streptococcus may have travelled via the auditory (or pharyngotympanic) tube into the middle ear, where it has caused inflammation which has spread to the mastoid cells. There is far less likelihood of the organism being transmitted from here because it is bottled up in the bone of the mastoid process, though it will continue to grow and form pus and unless this is released the infection may spread from the mastoid process into the cranial cavity. Again, the same organism may be causing an infection of a finger wound; provided this wound is kept covered by a germproof dressing, the organism cannot get out, but if it is left uncovered everything which the infected part touches may have organisms left on it.

If a patient has typhoid fever, the organism is at first present in the blood stream and for the first ten days the organism can be transmitted only by transfer of blood. Then the organism becomes localized in the lymph patches in the small intestine; and these break down and ulcerate, liberating the typhoid organisms into the stools, by which they can be transmitted to hands, bed pans, bed linen or the floor. Hence the importance of disinfecting the stools of a patient with typhoid fever before they are discharged, taking full isolation precautions, into the drainage system.

The second important factor in the problem of communicability is the length of time an organism capable of causing disease can live outside the human body. How long can the haemolytic streptococcus live on the sheets when it has been coughed there by the patient with tonsillitis or put there by the septic finger? How long can the typhoid bacillus live in the stools from the infected patient?

Bacteria vary enormously in the length of time that they can survive in unfavourable conditions and their communicability is profoundly affected by this. The organism of tuberculosis can live for many months protected by mucus in sputum, or in the dust away from sunlight, but the gonococcus, the organism causing gonorrhoea, is killed by half an hour in dry atmospheric air. Gonorrhoea can therefore be transmitted only by direct contact, from patient to patient, while tuberculosis can be caught by inhalation of dust from a room which has previously housed a tuberculosis patient.

Some organisms, like the haemolytic streptococcus, are relatively unexacting towards the tissues in which they grow, that is to say once they have invaded they can grow and multiply using any tissue in the body as a source of food, and growth will continue unless the organisms are killed by the defences of the body. Others are exacting in their requirements for growth, that is they are more selective and can find the necessary materials only in a particular type of tissue, such as brain tissue in the encephalitis group of viruses or the liver cells in infective hepatitis. If these exacting organisms do not reach the particular cells in which they can live, they will not produce disease and it is clear that the more exacting the organism, the more casualties there must be in its ranks to produce an infected patient.

The problem of communicability is thus extremely complex. Now that more is being learnt about the life history and the habits of pathogenic organisms and the course of disease, the hard and fast divisions of infectious, non-infectious, and contagious diseases are being modified. If the patient has a disease caused by a pathogenic organism, he is a danger to his fellow men if these organisms can get out and for as long as they are excreted whether intermittently or continuously. It is not possible to state categorically how long this will be in terms of days or weeks. If the organism is excreted in the urine or faeces, it is these excretions over which special care must be taken during their disposal. A patient with dysentery is excreting the pathogenic organism in his faeces, not by way of his nasal or respiratory secretions, so that no one in contact with him will be protected by wearing a mask. A patient with tuberculosis of the lungs has uninfected stools and no special care need be taken in the disposal of his faeces and urine, but a nurse attending him should wear a mask to prevent the inhalation of coughed-up organisms, and bed linen on which sputum may have fallen is potentially infected and should be kept separately. In both cases the nurse should wear a gown as the bed linen may be infected, and must wash her hands scrupulously before and after attending to the patient.

Healthy Carriers. Unfortunately the problem of infection is not as simple as the above paragraphs would suggest. Patients who have recovered from a disease and who are perfectly well may continue to excrete the pathogenic organism, which causes them no trouble but is a source of potential danger to the community. Clinical recovery should, as far as possible, be checked bacteriologically. In some people pathogenic organisms appear to live happily while producing in their host no symptoms at any time. Such persons are called carriers and they are unaware that they are a source of danger and may spread an infectious disease widely, for example the nurse from whose throat swab streptococci are grown. It appears that these organisms and their host live in harmony; the organisms do not invade but live on the mucous surfaces to be transmitted to another host where conditions may be more suitable for growth and invasion may occur.

It is for this reason that in some occupations involving the handling of food or water, in which pathogenic organisms can be transmitted with ease, the workers are bacteriologically investigated regularly to see if they are

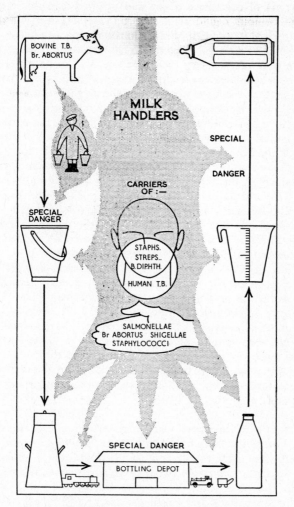

FIG. 8.—THE SPREAD OF INFECTION THROUGH MILK.

carriers of organisms which can be spread in this way, e.g. typhoid bacilli from the unwashed hands of an individual whose gall bladder harbours this organism.

Some organisms which cause characteristic diseases in one part of the body may be carried in quite another part, where they cause slight or no symptoms but from which they can be easily transmitted. A good example of this is the virus of poliomyelitis. It is a relatively common organism in children and young adults, causing a mild intestinal upset and malaise which is often called a 'cold' or 'influenza'. The doctor is often not sent for, so mild is the disease, but the organisms are passed in large numbers in the stools. They get on to the hands, thence to food and water. Only occasionally does this organism reach the nerve cells to cause the paralytic cases of classical infantile paralysis but in some instances even this infection could certainly be prevented by thorough washing of the hands before leaving the toilet.

The virus of infective hepatitis or epidemic jaundice is present in the stools of patients with infective hepatitis though there may be no intestinal symptoms.

Only by knowledge like this of the life history of pathogenic organisms is it possible to take reasonable precautions against infection. Much has yet to be learnt and much research which appeared at first to be only of academic interest is being found to have great practical importance in the study of the spread of infectious diseases.

Routes of Invasion. Organisms which cause disease may enter the body of the host by three different routes. They may enter the alimentary canal and cause disease there, e.g. the typhoid bacillus, and be thence absorbed into the circulation. They may be breathed into the respiratory tract and cause disease of the lungs, nasal cavity or some other part of the breathing apparatus;

for example, tuberculosis, pneumonia, the common cold, sore throats and many other conditions are spread in this way. They may pass through broken skin, and mucous membrane. Whole and healthy skin or mucous membrane will keep infection out, but if it is devitalized by bruising or by deficient diet, infection may pass through without there being any actual break.

These three routes of entry are spoken of as *ingestion*, i.e. the swallowing of infected food or water; *inhalation*, i.e. breathing in of infected air; *inoculation*, i.e. invasion through the skin or mucous membrane (Figs. 6–8).

Immunity

Immunity can be regarded as the result of the battle of two opposing forces, the pathogenic organism on the one hand and the host on the other hand. The result may be complete immunity, partial immunity or total absence of immunity, and the fight put up against the organism is termed the 'host's resistance'.

There is no such thing as a generalized immunity to all infectious diseases. Immunity is specific, that is it indicates the ability of the invaded to resist one particular invader; for example, the fact that we are told that a patient is immune to diphtheria gives us no information as to his immunity to any other unrelated disease, such as measles or tetanus.

In the first part of this chapter it was seen that the pathogenicity of an organism is a complex property which can be divided into three components:

(*a*) Invasiveness
     Destruction of vital cells
     Weakening vital structures
     Toxin formation
(*b*) Multiplication
(*c*) Communicability

The resistance of the host can therefore be divided into two parts; the prevention of invasion and the prevention of multiplication.

The Prevention of Invasion. The body is surrounded by organisms, both pathogenic and non-pathogenic, since they are present on everything we touch and eat and the air we breathe; therefore the skin and mucous surfaces must form the first line of defence.

The Skin. The skin has often been said to be impermeable to invasion by pathogenic organisms, but this is only a half-truth. The skin is not like a sheet of cellophane and the size of the organism has much to do with its ability to enter through the skin; certain of the minute viruses are capable of penetrating skin which appears to have no abrasions. The hair follicles and sweat glands harbour many organisms which it is impossible to remove in spite of the most meticulous treatment, and pathogenic organisms frequently invade from these sites. Axillary abscesses and beard infections are common results of such infection and are difficult to treat. Intact skin does, however, form a good barrier against many pathogenic bacteria, and sweat has a bactericidal action (pp. 29, 76).

Mucous Surfaces. In certain situations where the number of bacteria is high the surfaces are moistened with a mucous secretion to entrap the organisms until they can be removed; the nose, mouth and vagina are good examples of this. The damp dusting technique which can be used in the hospital ward is another example of trapping bacteria by moisture, as is the use of a good antiseptic furniture cream. Many new materials covering table tops and lockers can be washed daily or wiped over with a clean cloth soaked in antiseptic fluid.

Secretions. All organs in the body which are in contact with the external environment produce secretions. These are most appreciable in places where there is potentially the greatest danger of bacterial invasion. These secretions act in two ways:

(*a*) *By mechanical action.* Secretions of the bronchi entrap organisms and the flow of secretion is moved away from the alveoli by the action of the cilia on the bronchial walls. Tears also wash organisms away from the conjunctivae.

(*b*) *By chemical action of their constituents.* These secretions may be acid, like sweat, adult vaginal secretion and gastric juice, or contain fatty acids, like sweat, or be strongly alkaline, like bile. Abrupt changes from an acid to an alkaline environment are known, for example, to keep the bacterial flora of the alimentary canal in check. Tears contain an active antibacterial substance, lysozyme.

The Mechanical Arrangement of Structures. As air is inspired it is taken in at great force as if by a vacuum cleaner, and this air may contain many pathogenic organisms. The arrangement of the mucus-covered turbinate bones in the nose is such that the air impinges upon them, and bacteria stick to the mucous surfaces. The speed of flow of air is considerably reduced, due to the increasing area of the bronchial passages, with the result that by the time the air reaches the alveoli it is travelling very slowly and contains comparatively few organisms. The mucus, swept by the cilia up the air passages into the pharynx, is subsequently swallowed and many of the organisms are killed by the acid in the gastric juice.

The direction of the bronchi may have something to do with the localization of lung infections and the direction of the auditory tubes in infants may play a part in the greater frequency of middle ear infections in comparison with infections in adults.

Inside the body the mechanical arrangement of structures may also limit infection. Joint capsules, for instance, and tendon sheaths in the hand and foot do much to localize purulent material.

Causes of Resistance following Invasion. When a pathogenic organism manages to get through these barriers the course of events depends upon the body's other defences. At first the reaction of the body is the same for bacteria as it is for any other foreign body, it is the reaction of *inflammation*.

The signs of inflammation are: (1) heat; (2) redness; (3) swelling; (4) tenderness or pain. These signs depend upon a series of processes which are the same whether the foreign body is a staphyloccus, or a sterile splinter of wood.

Capillary dilatation results in an outpouring of fluid, white cells and some red cells from the vessels into the tissues. This outflow of fluid acts first of all by diluting the noxious agent and secondly by neutralizing or

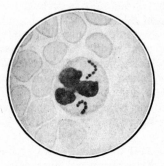

FIG. 9.—PHAGOCYTOSIS OF STREPTOCOCCI
BY POLYMORPHONUCLEAR LEUCOCYCTES.

inactivating any poisonous substances which may be produced by the invading organism. Plasma is able to do this because it contains antibacterial substances known as *antibodies*. These antibodies help to destroy the parasites which, once killed, are engulfed by the white cells and removed by the blood. This process is known as phagocytosis (Fig. 9). White cells which are destroyed by the infecting organism become pus cells, and pus is the accumulation of thousands of living and dead organisms, dead blood and tissue cells and liquefied tissue.

Some antibacterial substances present in normal plasma are non-specific; that is to say the substances act as well against staphylococci as against streptococci and are present to some extent in everyone. Their amount varies with the general health and nutrition of the patient and has some bearing on the different reaction of people to the same dose of an infective agent.

The invading organisms which have not been killed and engulfed by the white blood corpuscles are meanwhile growing and multiplying, deriving their food from the surrounding tissue and making from it more bacterial protoplasm. The bacterial protoplasm is complex since each organism is composed of many substances, such as protein, carbohydrate and lipid. These components are common to many organisms but the combination of substances is specific for or peculiar to any given organism, so that the protoplasm of one type of organism, whether minute like bacteria or large like the visible plants and animals, is different from the protoplasm of any other species of organism.

These substances formed by bacteria in the host tissues are foreign to the host and are called antigens. They stimulate the host to produce antibodies which are poured into the plasma to neutralize the effect of the antigens. Time is necessary for the production of these antibodies and they are not detectable in the patient's serum until 8 to 10 days after the start of an infection. The antibodies produced in response to an infection are specific, that is to say an attack of diphtheria causes the production of antibodies which will only neutralize diphtheria toxin or poison and will be of no use in combating a streptococcal infection.

Once an organism has invaded a patient's tissues it may multiply so rapidly that the patient succumbs before the specific antibodies have had time to be produced. Alternatively, antibodies may be produced, but in insufficient quantities to destroy the organism or neutralize its toxins, and the organism will overcome the specific resistance of the host; or antibodies may be produced in large quantities and succeed in killing the invading organism. The outcome of an infection is therefore the result of the battle between the forces of the organism and the resistance of the host in which the antibodies play a large part.

The antibodies, as we have seen, are not developed in large amounts until about 10 days after the onset of an infectious disease, and they last for a variable length of time. They are at their highest level in the serum immediately after recovery from the disease, and resistance to a particular infection is highest when the antibody level is highest. In some diseases, like measles, this level, once reached in response to an attack, declines very slowly so that more than one attack in a lifetime is extremely rare. In other diseases, like streptococcal infections, the antibody level falls relatively quickly, so that reinfection after months or even weeks is not uncommon.

Some infectious diseases, like influenza and the common cold, appear to confer very short-lived immunity, and it seems possible to have repeated attacks of diseases which are clinically identical. This may be due to the production of antibodies which are only short-lived, but it is probable that it is in part due to the fact that some organisms giving clinically similar disease are in fact antigenically different. The viruses producing the same clinical picture are composed of a different combination of proteins, carbohydrates and lipids and stimulate the production of different antibodies. The repeated common colds so often seen in the winter months may possibly be due to slightly different organisms.

Women who have produced antibodies as a result of infection pass these on to their babies through the placenta and in their milk. These antibodies do not last long, the baby is protected for the first few months of life only and then it begins to develop its own immunity because it can no longer depend upon the immunity of its mother.

Serum containing antibodies from convalescent patients has been used therapeutically for many years in the early stages of infection before a patient has had time to build up his own antibodies, or to prevent an attack when he has been exposed to infection; e.g. serum from adults who have recovered from measles (probably the infant's parents) can be used to protect a young baby who has been in contact with someone who has it. Antiserum is produced in large quantities by drug houses; horses are injected with a small dose of the causal organism or toxin producing the symptoms and then, after antibodies have had time to develop, the horses are bled and the serum used. The serum is tested for strength on animals and the strength is measured in units. Injection of serum containing large quantities of specific antibodies is known as passive immunization and it is used in diseases which are caused by organisms producing powerful toxins, such as diphtheria, tetanus and gas gangrene. The antibodies present in the horse serum act immediately by neutralizing the poisons circulating in the patient's blood stream. These antibodies are short-lived, however, and passive immunization is used to prevent an attack after contact with the disease, or is used repeatedly once a disease has developed until the patient has had the time and strength to produce his own. Thus a patient who might by the nature of his wound be suspected of having incurred the risk of infection by the tetanus bacillus may be given on admission a massive dose of antitetanus serum, or a booster dose of tetanus toxoid if he has already been immunized. This is because the earlier the injection is given, the greater the chance of recovery.

It has been found possible to stimulate, artificially, the production of specific antibodies in patients by the process of active immunization, so that the antibodies are produced without the patient having the disease. This is now done on a large scale in the immunization against diphtheria, typhoid, yellow fever and tetanus, to mention only a few, and in horses as already stated in order to produce the serum for passive immunization. Briefly this is made possible by altering the causative organism, by heating, diluting or treating with chemicals so that it is no longer pathogenic but is still antigenic, that is to say capable of stimulating antibody formation. Another method of stimulating immunity is by injecting a closely related but harmless organism, some of whose antigens are similar to those of the pathogenic organism, e.g. the lymph containing the vaccinia of cowpox is used to inoculate people against smallpox.

Immunity may be of two kinds; *inherent* and *acquired*. Acquired immunity to a disease can be differentiated from inherent immunity in that it is associated with detectable specific antibodies in the serum while inherent immunity is not.

Acquired Immunity. Acquired immunity is associated with the presence of specific circulating antibodies

TYPES OF IMMUNITY

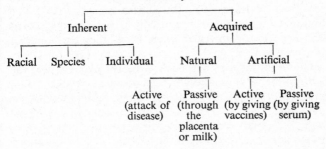

Immunity

Inherent | Acquired

Racial   Species   Individual   Natural   Artificial

Active (attack of disease)   Passive (through the placenta or milk)   Active (by giving vaccines)   Passive (by giving serum)

which may have developed naturally as a result of an attack of the disease, or artificially by active immunization. They may on the other hand have been formed in some other person or animal and been actually transferred to the patient through the placenta or by injection of antiserum.

The detection of antibodies in the serum of a patient is useful in diagnosis. Their presence, provided the patient has not been immunized either actively or passively, means that the specific antigen must be stimulating their production. If it can be shown that a patient is producing typhoid antibodies then typhoid organisms must be present, causing these antibodies to be made. The diagnosis of typhoid fever can therefore be made, though the organism was not isolated. It may be 8 to 14 days before the antibodies can be demonstrated, so that a diagnosis dependent upon this method is necessarily delayed.

Inherent Immunity. Inherent immunity is difficult to assess, and is bound up with the metabolic requirements of the organism and the way of life of the host. It probably does not often occur.

Racial immunity is usually only relative and complete

racial immunity is very rare. In man some races are known to be susceptible and others relatively immune to certain diseases, e.g. the Jewish race is said to be immune to tuberculosis and this is in part dependent upon the nutrition, cleanliness, economics and genetics of the race.

The immunity of a species is more clear cut but the reason for it is unknown. Certain diseases like poliomyelitis, syphilis and leprosy, occur spontaneously in man and can be transmitted to experimental animals only with the greatest difficulty. Other diseases, like tuberculosis, anthrax and psittacosis, occur spontaneously in both man and animals. Those diseases limited to one species are in the main those caused by organisms which are very exacting in their growth requirements, and it is probable that the required conditions for growth are met with only in that one species.

Individual immunity is a problem of great complexity which cannot be gone into here. In a crowd the variation in response to a given infection is mainly due to previously acquired immunity and is not due to an inherent immunity at all. The difference in response given by adults and children reflects a physiological change in certain tissues. For instance the anatomy of the auditory tube and middle ear in infants makes invasion of pathogenic organisms easier in them than in adults. The vagina at puberty produces an acid secretion which is bactericidal. Nutrition, fatigue, exposure to cold and damp and even emotional states, all have a bearing on the individual's response to infection.

5 THE MICROSCOPE

Since bacteria are microscopic in size, it is important for the nurse to have some working knowledge of the microscope, the instrument which plays such an important part in their study. A microscope consists essentially of two lenses, the objective and the eyepiece. These are separated and held in correct relative position by the body tube, the eyepiece being fitted into the upper end and the objective screwed to the lower; together they form the combined optical unit, which is fixed to a stand on which it can be raised or lowered by means of coarse and fine adjustment, so that the optical point is focused on the slide which is being examined (Fig. 10).

The slide holding the specimen is carried by a stage fixed to the stand below the body tube. This stage is at right angles to the optical axis of the body tube and may be fitted with a mechanical arrangement permitting precise movement of the specimen. This movement can be measured on a scale on the sides of the stage. The stage has an aperture in the centre to allow light rays to be reflected from a concave mirror below it through the slide into the body tube and to the eye of the observer.

Beneath the stage is another optical unit, the substage condenser, with a diaphragm, and a centring device to ensure proper illumination of the field that is being observed. It is not essential when using lower degrees of magnification, but when the higher degrees necessary to make microorganisms visible are used a condenser is required. It consists essentially of a lens to focus light

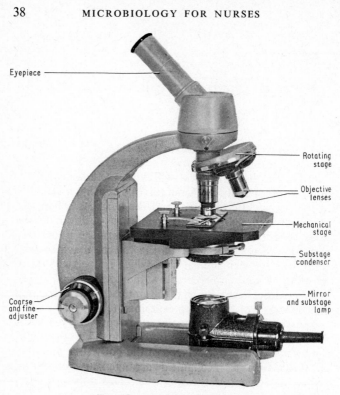

FIG. 10. A MODERN MICROSCOPE

on the specimen being examined and a diaphragm, like the iris of the eye, which can be adjusted to control the amount of light which reaches the field being viewed, since too high a concentration of light blinds, and too little also makes sight impossible.

Light, either daylight or artificial light, is directed on to the mirror beneath the stage, the latter being adjusted to the right angle to deflect the light rays on to the substage condenser. This focuses the light on the object under examination. Magnification of the specimen is brought about by the objective and the eyepiece; each microscope has a number of different objectives and eyepieces which give varying degrees of magnification, from 60 to 800 times the size of the object viewed. Magnification by the objective is focused by means of coarse and fine adjustment and results in a real, primary, enlarged and inverted image at its focal point in the tube. This real image is further magnified by the eyepiece, which gives a virtual, secondary image which the eye sees.

Magnification of an object therefore depends on three things:

(1) The focal length of the objective. This may be defined as the distance from the lens at which parallel rays are brought together; the more convex the lens, the shorter the focal length.

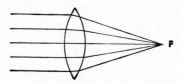

FIG. 11.—A CONVEX LENS, SHOWING HOW PARALLEL LIGHT RAYS ARE BROUGHT TO A FOCUS AT POINT F.

(2) The magnifying power of the eyepiece.
(3) The distance between the lens system of the objective and the image.

Lenses used in bacteriological work are those of high magnification and thus have short focal lengths; therefore the objective, when focused, is very close to the specimen. Because it is so close care is needed in adjusting the focus, since it is easy for the inexperienced, by turning the adjustment screws in the wrong direction, to hit the slide with the objective and break it. Light deflected by the mirror has to pass through air, the condenser, air, the glass slide, and air again before entering the optical system of the microscope. When rays travel from air to glass they are bent towards the normal, and when emerging into the air again they are bent away from the normal; in this process much valuable light is lost. In

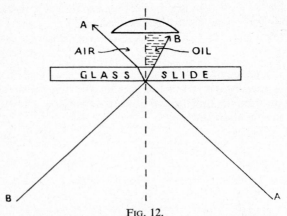

FIG. 12.
THE PATHS OF LIGHT RAYS THROUGH A GLASS SLIDE.

When the marginal rays (AA) pass through air they are bent so much that they do not reach the lens. If an oil-immersion lens is used, with oil of the same refractive index as glass, the rays (BB) are not bent so much.

order to avoid this loss oil of the same refractive index as glass (i.e. oil through which light travels at the same rate and therefore in the same line as through glass, so that no bending of the light rays occurs) is used to fill the space between the slide and the lens and prevent deviation when high magnification is being used. The short focus lens giving high degrees of magnification is therefore called the oil-immersion lens. Objectives are also known by the focal length of their lenses. Common examples are the 16 mm ($\frac{2}{3}$ in.), 4 mm ($\frac{1}{6}$ in.) and 2 mm ($\frac{1}{12}$ in.) objectives, also known by their initial magnifying powers, $\times$ 10, $\times$ 40, $\times$ 100 respectively. For examining bacteria the $\frac{1}{12}$ in. objective is generally used, and this is an oil-immersion lens. Many microscopes are made with a rotating nose piece at the lower end of the body tube which will carry three objectives at the same time. This is convenient because it enables the viewer to examine a specimen first under lower magnification and then, by turning the nose piece, to bring the stronger objective into line with the body tube in order to obtain higher magnification without unscrewing and putting away the one already used.

The eyepieces are numbered according to their strength. The lower numbers (e.g. 1 to 6) give less magnification and the higher numbers (e.g. 6 to 10) give greater magnification. The eyepiece fits exactly into the tube and the whole tube is moved gently up or down until the focus is perfect and the image is seen in clearly defined outlines. A blurred picture means that the focus needs adjustment. The eyepiece has a milled edge to make it easy to insert and remove.

The nurse should know how to use a microscope intelligently, although she need not memorize the facts concerning it. When using it for the first time, it is helpful to look at objects that can be seen with the naked eye, such as a hair, or a fine strand of cotton or wool, and then at a drop of milk or blood, under different objectives, and thus gain an idea of the degree of magnification that the microscope gives. After use, the parts should be cleaned, as necessary, and the instrument, which is expensive and difficult to replace, should be put carefully away.

To examine a slide, first place the microscope in position facing the source of light being used and adjust the mirror to reflect a good light into the body tube. Then place the slide on the stage, with the specimen to be examined below the objective. Next lower the objective close to the slide watching it from the side. Then with the eye close to the eyepiece, turn the coarse adjustment slowly to raise the body tube till the slide comes into focus. Finally turn the fine adjustment slowly till the focus is perfect and the object being examined is seen clearly. Because of differences in vision between individuals especially persons who are definitely short- or long-sighted, the focus may need adjustment for different persons, especially when high degrees of magnification are being used. In carrying out adjustment by raising the body tube slowly, the danger of breaking slides by striking them with the objective is avoided: this is specially important, when using high degrees of magnification with an oil-immersion lens, as the objective is very close to the slide. It is not necessary to close or cover the eye that is not being used as with practice it becomes easy to concentrate on the picture seen by the eye looking down the microscope and ignore what is seen by the other eye.

DIAGNOSTIC MICROBIOLOGY
6 AND PRACTICAL
DEMONSTRATIONS

DIAGNOSTIC microbiology is the province of the micro-biologist, but it is necessary for the nurse to know some of the processes involved if the best use of the laboratory is to be made, and both its scope and its limitations must be recognized.

Broadly speaking microbiological diagnosis of an infectious disease rests on:

1. Recovery of the causative organism from infected material.
2. Demonstration of antibodies to a pathogenic organism in the patient's serum.

The Choice of Material for Isolation of the Causative Organism

As a general rule the more material sent for investigation the greater the chance of isolating the causative organism. Samples of secretions likely to contain the pathogenic organism should be collected before antibiotic treatment has begun or immediately before the next dose is given. These samples should be put in a sterile container, adequately labelled and sent to the laboratory immediately.

Certain microbiological investigations have become routine procedures:

Nose and Throat Swabs. Swabs from the nose and

throat are usually taken together, one swab for both tonsils and one for both nostrils; organisms causing sore throats are frequently carried in the nose and failure to take nose swabs may mean that the organisms here are missed.

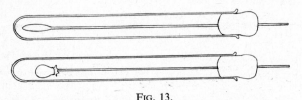

FIG. 13.
(*Above*) A sterile swab.
(*Below*) A sterile swab wrapped in cellophane.

The patient is placed facing a strong source of light and the tongue is depressed. The swab should never be removed from its sterile tube until everything is ready for taking the specimen. When taking a throat swab care should be taken to avoid touching the mouth or tongue with the swab, which should be pressed into the tonsils or tonsillar bed in an effort to squeeze out infected material from the crypts. When taking nasal swabs it is important to ensure that the swab reaches as far back as possible on each side; this can usually be done by tilting the patient's head back and using a gentle twisting movement.

With babies and very young children wooden swab sticks are often too large to get into the nostrils and many hospitals supply fine wire swabholders covered with a tiny wisp of cotton wool. Care is needed to avoid damage to the delicate mucous membranes with these swabs and some doctors prefer to take these specimens personally. Swabs should be replaced in the sterile containers immediately, to avoid contamination with air organisms.

Ear Swabs. The same type of swab stick is used for ear swabs as for nose and throat swabs, and care should be taken that no antibiotics or other chemotherapeutic or antiseptic material has been used in the ear within three hours of taking the swab.

Wound Swabs. Wound swabs are usually taken when a dressing is being changed; the same type of swab stick is used as for ear, nose and throat swabs.

Puncture Fluids. Large quantities of material for microbiological investigation are usually taken by syringe and may be transferred directly from this syringe to a sterile bottle. The fluids taken include pleural fluid, peritoneal fluid and cerebrospinal fluid. Fluids requiring a cell count should be put into two sterile bottles appropriately labelled; the second one should be used for the count, since the first may contain extraneous blood cells introduced into the syringe as it went through the tissues.

Sputum. The sputum is never free from organisms since the bronchi and alveoli are in direct contact with unsterile air. It is therefore unnecessary to collect specimens into sterilized containers, but these should be clean; in many laboratories wax cartons are used which can be burned after the investigation is complete. No disinfectant should be put in sputum pots which are to be sent for microbiological investigation.

Care should be taken that the material sent for investigation is in fact sputum and not saliva. Patients who have difficulty in bringing up phlegm should be encouraged to cough first thing in the morning. Patients with coughs usually have mucopurulent, or purulent flecks in the specimen. The specimen should be as large as possible and it is better to wait until an adequate specimen can be produced than to waste laboratory time on minute specimens of saliva. When the specimen has been coughed up the bacterial population alters in proportion rapidly; it is therefore important that the specimen should be sent to the laboratory immediately.

Specimens of Sputum in Cases of Tuberculosis. The tubercle bacillus, *Mycobacterium tuberculosis*, may sometimes be thinly distributed in the sputum and a large quantity of material must therefore be submitted. The bacillus is most likely to be present in the purulent flecks. It is particularly important in tuberculosis to submit adequate specimens as the organisms may be seen in direct films from the sputum. It is also necessary to make cultures. It is usual to send three specimens of sputum taken on different days when looking for the tubercle bacillus; the results may not be available for 6 weeks or even longer, because cultures grow slowly. It may also be necessary to inject the material into guinea pigs to see whether they contract the disease before making a diagnosis (p. 60).

Urine. Specimens of urine should normally be taken in the early morning when the urine has accumulated in the bladder over night: all specimens from one patient are then roughly comparable. If they are taken at other times the urine may sometimes be diluted due to a high fluid intake. Early morning specimens are not of course possible in out-patient clinics, but they should be the rule for in-patients. In examination for tubercle bacilli in the urine, where the organisms are likely to be very scanty, the whole of the specimen should be sent in a sterile bottle.

Specimens of urine from male patients should be 'mid-stream specimens', that is to say, specimens taken after the skin surrounding the urethral meatus has been cleansed with an antiseptic, and the first part of the urine discarded. This avoids contamination of the specimen with organisms normally present on the skin.

A sterile catheter specimen of urine from female patients for bacteriological examination may still be required. In most cases, however, a mid-stream specimen is preferred, and various methods have been evolved to avoid contamination; again the first urine passed is discarded. When a catheter specimen is necessary the surrounding skin and vulva is carefully cleansed before introduction of the catheter and the part of the catheter which enters the bladder and urethra should not touch any external part before it enters the urethra, nor be touched with ungloved hands. Should contamination occur the catheter must be discarded.

Faeces. Specimens of stools for examination should be sent in clean but unsterile cartons which may be subsequently burnt. Some bacteriologists prefer rectal swabs for the detection of the organisms causing food poisoning or dysentery. These swabs are of the same type as those used for wounds and the nose and throat, and care should be taken to pass the swab through the anus right into the rectum. It is advisable to send a specimen of stool as well if this is available so that the amount of pus, blood and mucus and the consistency of the specimen can then be seen.

Specimens of Stools for Worms. This is conveniently mentioned here.

Tapeworms. Segments of tapeworm can be seen with ease in any specimen of stool and the worm will continue to grow and shed segments unless the head is dislodged; it is therefore important to search for this in every specimen passed by the patient after treatment. Stool specimens should be strained through fine black material under a running tap, the tapeworm segments will be

retained and can be sent to the laboratory for identification of the species and for confirmation of the presence
of the head.

Ova. Many intestinal worms shed their ova into the
faeces; they can only be seen microscopically and a fresh
specimen of stool should be sent to the laboratory in a
waxed carton. Threadworms lay their ova on the anal
skin; swabs of this area should therefore be taken as the
ova will not be seen in stool specimens.

Swabs for taking specimens from the anal mucosa are
glass rods covered at the end with cellophane paper and
sterilized in glass tubes (Fig. 13, p. 44).

Specimens of Stool for Amoebae. It is also convenient
to mention here the collection of specimens of stool for
examination for amoeba. The parasites of amoebic
dysentery, *Entamoeba histolytica,* exist in a free-living
motile form and in the form of non-motile cysts. Both
forms are characteristic in their fresh state and a diagnosis
of amoebic dysentery can be made from a fresh specimen
of stool. The free-living form, however, becomes non-
motile very easily in older specimens when the temperature has fallen, and both forms are more difficult to
recognize when they are dead. It is therefore essential
that specimens of stool for amoebae should be brought
to the laboratory as soon as they are taken and should be
looked at immediately. Many specimens may be
necessary before the amoebae are seen.

Eye Swabs. Either a wire loop or cotton wool-covered
wooden stick should be used (Fig. 13, p. 44). Rub gently
over the conjunctiva in the lower conjunctival sac, taking
care to hold the swab parallel to the cornea and to avoid
contamination by touching the lids.

Purulent conjunctivitis in babies may be due to the
gonococcus, which is a very delicate organism and may

be killed if the swabs are allowed to dry or get cold. In some hospitals it is a routine procedure in cases of purulent conjunctivitis, to take two swabs. One of these swabs is broken into a bottle of transport medium, which can be kept in the ward ready for use and will prevent the delicate organisms from dying; the other swab can be sent to the laboratory together with this bottle so that direct films of the pus can be stained. In this way swabs taken at any time of the day or night will come to no harm and treatment can begin as soon as they have been taken.

Vaginal Swabs. Special curved swabs should be used and the specimens should be taken from as high in the vaginal vault as possible after introduction of a speculum to separate the walls. If a *Trichomonas* infection is suspected an additional swab should be sent in normal saline which may be put into the bottom of the swab tube. These swabs should be taken to the laboratory immediately. Specimens may also be taken with a teated pipette contained in a test tube.

Blood Cultures. Samples of blood are usually taken by the medical officer and are used for direct isolation of a pathogenic organism in a case of septicaemia, and for detection of antibodies in the serum; in either case the specimens should be taken with sterile precautions; a dry, sterile syringe is used.

Success or failure in isolating organisms present in the blood stream is largely dependent upon taking the specimen at the right time and putting it into suitable medium for cultivation, and in this the nursing staff can give valuable assistance.

The clinician will tell the microbiologist what organism he thinks may be present, the microbiologist will choose the correct medium, and the blood is put directly into one or more bottles of this fluid. Organisms are most likely to be present in the blood stream in the greatest number when the temperature is at its highest, so that the most favourable time for taking a blood culture is at the peak of the temperature. The ward sister's knowledge of the patient's previous temperature range will help in predicting when this is likely to be, and it is her duty to keep a watch on his temperature and inform the medical officer or the laboratory when this is rising. With all requests for blood cultures certain information should be sent to the laboratory:

1. The time the blood culture was taken and the patient's temperature at that time.
2. The length of time the patient has been ill.
3. Any inflammatory lesions the patient may have, e.g. pneumonia, septic wound, urinary infection and the microbiology of these lesions if known.
4. Any chemotherapeutic treatment the patient may be having, and when he had his last dose. (Chemotherapeutic drugs for this purpose would include antibiotics.)

Serum for detection of antibodies. For this investigation 10 ml of blood should be taken into a dry tube or bottle containing no anticoagulant, and allowed to clot.

As previously noted, specific antibodies do not appear in the serum for several days. It is the usual procedure to take blood at the beginning of a disease and then again after 10 days; the specimens are examined together in the laboratory. An increase in the number of antibodies in the second specimen will be an indication of continued stimulation by the organism which must therefore be present in the patient. By comparing two specimens more information is gained, although single samples are sometimes helpful.

It is important that samples are accompanied by full details of:

(a) The clinical history
(b) The length of time the patient has been ill
(c) Any history of a previous attack of the disease, with dates
(d) Any history of immunization against typhoid fever

Isolation of the Causative Organism from Infected Material

The microbiologist identifies an organism in material which is sent to him by a number of tests which have been designed to tell him a series of facts:

(1) Morphology or size and shape of the organism and its staining properties
(2) Condition of growth
(3) Cultural characteristics
(4) Biochemical tests
(5) Resistance
(6) Serological tests
(7) Pathogenicity tests in experimental animals

Morphology of the Organism

The organisms present in any specimen sent to the microbiologist are examined to determine their size, shape and other specific characteristics (pp. 6, 8). They may be from 0·3 μ to 14 μ in length (1 $\mu = \frac{1}{1000}$ mm). They may be round, rod-shaped or spiral. They may grow in pairs, in clusters or in chains, and a given culture may contain organisms of irregular size and shape. They may possess flagella or may contain spores. To make them readily visible they are stained with various dyes in different ways to distinguish them according to the effects of various staining processes.

Staining. The bacterial kingdom can be roughly divided into two by the action of a staining technique called *Gram's method*, which consists of staining the cells with a basic dye, methyl violet, and afterwards treating with iodine. The excess stain is then washed off with alcohol or acetone, until no more can be removed. The organisms are subsequently counterstained with a contrasting coloured dye, e.g. carbol fuchsin. Gram positive organisms are those which retain the methyl violet and appear purple under the microscope. Gram negative ones are those which do not retain the dye and are stained pale pink by the counterstain. Hence bacteria are divided into Gram positive and Gram negative groups and this grouping, together with the bacterial shape, cocci, bacilli or very short ovoid organisms called coccobacilli, gives the bacteriologist a start in his identification.

The tubercle bacillus (*Mycobacterium tuberculosis*) and related organisms are stained only with difficulty by Gram's stain, but can be stained by using hot, strong carbol fuchsin, which stain is impossible to remove with acid and alcohol. This is the basis of the *Ziehl-Neelsen* stain and the organisms so stained are said to be 'acid-alcohol fast'.

Organisms which are able to move by means of flagella or hairlike structures which may be placed in various positions on the bacterial body can be stained by special techniques only. The spirochaetes such as *Treponema pallidum*, the organism responsible for syphilis, are capable of movement by bending their spiral bodies and the rate and character of the movement is characteristic.

Dark staining areas may be seen in some organisms. These may be demonstrated by various stains and their presence or absence is helpful. Some organisms such as the pneumococcus, can produce a sticky material which surrounds the organism like a capsule.

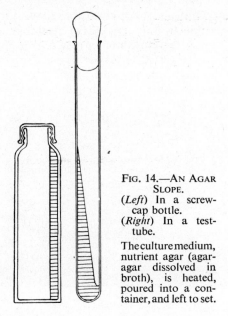

FIG. 14.—AN AGAR SLOPE.
(*Left*) In a screw-cap bottle.
(*Right*) In a test-tube.

The culture medium, nutrient agar (agar-agar dissolved in broth), is heated, poured into a container, and left to set.

Condition of Growth

It is the usual procedure, when endeavouring to isolate an organism, to put infected material into a mixture containing nutriment which is suitable to encourage the growth of likely organisms. The foodstuffs are called 'culture media' and many have a meat infusion, like clear soup, as a basis, which is put into sterile bottles; a swab previously dipped in infected material is broken into one of these. The meat infusion may be mixed with hot melted agar-agar, poured into flat glass dishes called Petri dishes or into test tubes, and allowed to set. Infected material is spread on to the surface using a fine wire loop (p. 48).

When agar is the culture medium that is used the plate

is incubated with the lid downward to prevent the water of condensation from falling on the medium.

To encourage the growth of various organisms certain other substances can be added to this basic medium. For example, amino-acids, proteins in the form of serum, plasma or whole blood, or vitamins. It is also possible by

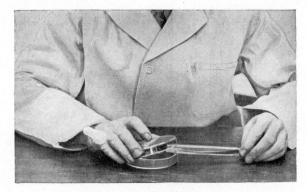

FIG. 15.—POURING A PLATE.

Pouring liquid culture medium into a Petri dish. So as to prevent the entry of bacteria from the air the lid of the dish is lifted at one side only just sufficiently to allow the tube to be introduced.

the use of selective media to inhibit the growth of certain organisms. Selective media are those which contain substances which are known to inhibit certain organisms, or groups of organisms.

An example of this is the addition of gentian violet to an agar plate, which will inhibit the growth of a staphylococcus. If an organism which is suspected of being a staphylococcus from its morphology fails to grow on a medium containing gentian violet, this is confirmatory evidence of its being a staphylococcus.

Selective media are also useful in the detection of

PLATE II

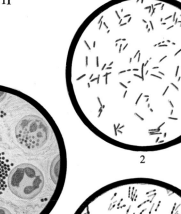

2

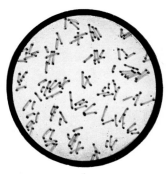

1

1. STAPHYLOCOCCI IN PUS.

2. *C. DIPHTHERIAE*. FILM
STAINED BY GRAM'S METHOD.

3. *C. DIPHTHERIAE*. FILM
STAINED WITH METHYLENE
BLUE.

4. *C. DIPHTHERIAE*. FILM
STAINED BY NEISSER'S METHOD.

3

4

pathogenic organisms from material such as stools and throat swabs, both of which are normally full of organisms. If unselective enriched media are used, the normal non-pathogenic organisms may overgrow the sparse pathogens and make their detection difficult. In practice there are now selective media for the majority of species and certain media have become routine for primary inoculation of material from most sites.

Cultural Characteristics

In order to ascertain the cultural characteristics of an organism, infected material is introduced into suitable fluid and solid media. On the latter it is spread thinly over the whole plate with a wire loop, which is sterilized in a flame before and after use. The inoculated media are then put into incubators adjusted to a constant temperature. In medical microbiology 37° C (98·4° F) is the temperature of primary incubation, because the majority of human pathogens have this as their optimum temperature. After isolation, however, the temperature range at which an organism can grow is of much diagnostic importance (Fig. 16).

Many organisms, such as the staphylococcus or the diphtheria bacillus, grow best in an atmosphere containing oxygen; they grow well therefore in air and are said to be aerobic organisms. Some, such as the meningococcus, the organism causing cerebrospinal fever, grow best in an atmosphere containing carbon dioxide, and for isolation of this organism from a case of meningitis the inoculated plates are put into a tin which contains 5% carbon dioxide and are put in the incubator. Other organisms, such as *Clostridium tetani*, cannot grow where there is free oxygen, and to grow these organisms conditions must be made anaerobic by placing the plates in a tin or jar, evacuating the air and replacing it with hydrogen. These are strictly anaerobic organisms, but there are some that are aerobes, although facultatively anaerobic, that is to say they are equipped with enzymes which bring about both aerobic and anaerobic respiration. Organisms such as streptococci fall into this group.

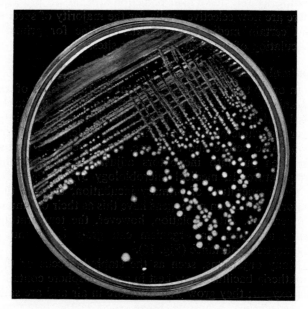

FIG. 16.

COLONIES ON A PLATE SPREAD BY THE METHOD OF
PARALLEL STREAKS.

A small portion of the material to be examined is spread over the surface by successive parallel strokes of a wire loop.

It is usual to leave the plates undisturbed in the incubator for 18 to 24 hours before looking for growth. Some organisms grow slowly and often no growth may be visible to the naked eye at this time. With other organisms, along the lines of inoculation there will be heaped colonies of growing organisms, ranging from 0·1 mm to 4 mm in size. These colonies, each containing many single organisms which have developed by division of the initial ones put on with the loop, are characteristic

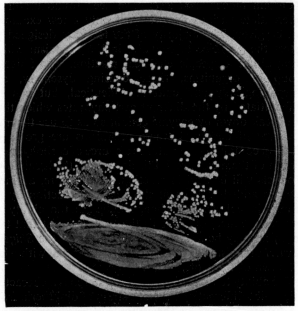

FIG. 17.

COLONIES ON A PLATE INOCULATED BY SPREADING.

A drop of the material is rubbed over a small portion of the surface by means of a wire spreader measuring 3 to 4 cm across. The spreader is then lifted and rubbed over a fresh area.

for the species. Their size, shape, colour, consistency and effect on the surrounding medium are all of importance. Instead of isolated colonies the organisms may have spread in a film all over the plate; organisms which do this are those which are highly motile, that is capable of movement in the thin film of water which covers the surface of the plate.

Biochemical Tests

Certain biochemical tests have been found useful to differentiate various bacteria, but only a few examples can be given. The majority of the tests are designed to detect the presence of enzymes in the organism which bring about a specific chemical reaction. The Shigella group of organisms, those causing dysentery, are morphologically and culturally identical, but can be differentiated by the different carbohydrates which they can break down by enzyme action, so as to use them as a source of energy. If these organisms are grown in medium containing mannitol as a source of carbohydrate, certain of them can break this down, and the breakdown products will be acid in reaction. If, therefore, an indicator is added which will show acid production by its change in colour, this change indicates the ability to ferment the alcohol and tells the bacteriologist that this organism may be *Shigella sonnei*, or one of the *Shigella flexneri* organisms, if other reactions also fit in with what is known of these organisms.

The ability to break down and use starch is a characteristic which differentiates the one strain of diphtheria from the other members of the genus *Corynebacterium*, and is a useful differentiating test. The ability to form indole in a medium containing tryptophan is a characteristic of many non-pathogenic members of the colon group of organisms. There are many other examples used diagnostically, all reflecting a fundamental metabolic process which has by experience been found useful in differentiating one organism from another.

Resistance

The resistance of an organism to temperature, drying,

acid, antiseptics, dyes, chemotherapeutic agents and antibodies, is a help in diagnosis as well as a help in treatment and prevention of spread. As we have already seen, those organisms which have not the power of forming spores are relatively less resistant to heat than the spore-bearing organisms. Some haemolytic streptococci will be killed if kept at 60° C for 30 minutes; *Clostridium botulinum* will stand at least 100° C for 60 minutes.

Closely related organisms, such as various kinds of streptococci, may be differentiated by a heat resistance test, the latter withstanding 60° C for 30 minutes, and this forms a useful diagnostic test.

Some organisms are sensitive to bile; a pneumococcus may be differentiated from a viridans type of streptococcus by tests making use of this principle.

It has already been mentioned that staphylococci are sensitive to gentian violet. The sensitivity of various organisms to the antibiotics, although it may be of value in differentiating strains, is of more value as a guide to therapy.

Serology

An organism isolated from infected material contains numerous antigens; if these are mixed with serum containing known specific antibodies prepared by injection of a known organism into an experimental animal, and the unknown organism reacts with the specific antiserum, the antigens in the unknown organism must be the same as or closely related to those which were used to immunize the experimental animal. Antigen–antibody reactions are used a great deal in bacteriology, the union of antigen with antibody being associated with an altered physical state of the mixture such as a clumping of red blood cells, which enables it to be seen. Use is also made of these reactions, as we have seen before, in detecting unknown antibodies in the patient's serum, the serum being mixed with known organisms acting as antigens. This principle forms the basis of the Wassermann test for syphilis and the Widal test for enteric fever (Figs. 18 and 19).

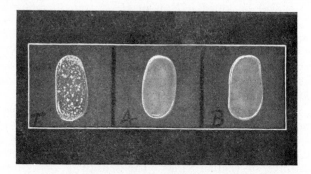

FIG. 18.—SLIDE AGGLUTINATION SEEN BY NAKED EYE.

A culture of bacteria from a suspected typhoid carrier has been mixed with drops of antisera prepared against *Salmonella typhi* (T), *Salm. paratyphi* (A), and *Salm. paratyphi* (B). It has been agglutinated by T but not by A or B. Therefore the organism is identified as the typhoid bacillus.

Inoculation of Infected Material into Laboratory Animals

Some infectious agents cannot be cultured on artificial media, and their presence can only be detected by producing the disease in an experimental animal which is known to be susceptible. Tissues from the animal may show changes typical of the disease. For example, when tubercle bacilli cannot be found in the urine, tuberculosis may sometimes be produced in a guinea pig by injection with some of the fluid.

The tubercle bacillus is similar morphologically to non-pathogenic members of the same genus, and in some cases can only be differentiated from the non-pathogenic members of the genus by inoculation into laboratory animals. Pathogenic tubercle bacilli are identified by the typical lesions which they produce, both macroscopically and microscopically.

Injection of infected material into two experimental animals, one of which has been protected previously by

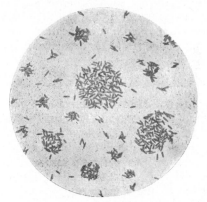

FIG. 19.—AGGLUTINATION AS SEEN UNDER THE MICROSCOPE.

a specific antiserum, is also used as a method of diagnosing disease. Animal protection experiments are used to a certain extent in virus diagnosis.

Certain strains of pathogenic organisms, such as diphtheria bacilli, produce powerful exotoxins or poisons which are responsible for much of the clinical picture of diphtheria. Some strains of diphtheria bacilli, however, though otherwise identical with these toxin-producers, produce no toxin, and are, therefore, harmless. Toxin-producing strains can be identified by their pathogenicity to guinea pigs.

These are the means, then, by which the bacteriologist is able to identify organisms present in the material which is sent to him, but it will be obvious that this identification is bound to take time. In rare cases the organisms can be seen in direct films of the material and their appearance will be diagnostic. More commonly 18 hours is necessary for the organisms to be grown on media and only then can the various differential tests be applied.

In specimens taken from sites which are normally inhabited by organisms, such as the respiratory tract, the stools, and lesions involving the skin, the bacterial flora will be mixed and before identification can begin the organisms must be separated and isolated in pure culture.

The Demonstration of Antibodies in Patients' Serum

The diagnosis of infectious disease by demonstrating the presence of antibodies in the patient's serum is dealt with under Immunity in Chapter 4; it is as well to note that the inference to be drawn from the presence of specific antibodies in a patient's serum is limited. All that can be deduced is that the patient has at some time been subjected to the specific antigen under test. This may have been a previous infection or subclinical infection of the disease; it may have been active immunization against the disease, or it may have been an attack of a closely related disease, the causative organism of which contains a common antigen; or it may be a present attack of the disease. A present attack of the disease is best diagnosed by taking repeated samples of serum and showing that these contain an increase in antibody content or 'titre'.

Hypersensitivity Tests suggesting a Previous Dose of a Pathogenic Organism

Foreign proteins, as already stated, when injected into animals or people, act as antigens. The response of a patient to the first dose of an antigen differs from his response to the second and subsequent doses. This difference is more marked in some subjects than others and with some antigens than with others.

When the first dose of antigens causes a marked difference in reaction, as with tuberculosis, the patient is said to be 'sensitized' to that antigen, following the primary dose. This sensitivity, or altered reaction, can be demonstrated by the marked erythematous reaction with induration which occurs when the antigen is injected intradermally into a patient who has previously had a dose of the antigen, in contrast to the absence of this reaction in the unsensitized patient who has never encountered the antigen.

This reaction of sensitivity is the basis of the Mantoux reaction and patch test in tuberculosis, and the Casoni test in hydatid disease. A positive reaction does not necessarily mean that the patient has the active disease at the time of the test, but that he has at some previous date had a dose of the antigen. The diagnostic value of a positive Mantoux test is therefore limited. Many people have a primary dose of tuberculosis in their childhood or adolescence, which they overcome without difficulty and with no clinical symptoms, and the majority of adults are therefore Mantoux positive. The younger the child, however, the more significance can be placed on a positive test, because the child has had less time to overcome the primary infection, and great care should be taken to ascertain that the infection has been arrested.

Non-specific Tests

There are certain tests which have been found by experience to be positive in certain diseases, although the reasons are unknown. These tests are mainly antigen–antibody reactions. The patient's serum in certain diseases contains an antibody which reacts with an antigen which did not stimulate its production, that is to say, one other than the infecting agent. It is probable that this infecting agent and the test antigen are, however, chemically and antigenically related. This happens in some circumstances with the *Salmonella* group of diseases.

Weil-Felix Reaction. An attack of typhus stimulates the production of antibodies which react with a certain strain of a *Proteus* organism, and in this test the *Proteus* organism is used as the antigen. More specific tests, using the typhus rickettsia itself, are replacing this test.

Cold Agglutinins. The infective agent or agents responsible for virus pneumonia have never been isolated, so that specific antigen–antibody reactions are not possible. It has been shown, however, that certain patients with this disease develop in their serum antibodies which agglutinate human group O cells at a low temperature. This is of some help in diagnosis.

There are many examples, too numerous to mention, of non-specific serological tests used in diagnosis of past or present infectious diseases, and as more is known of the antigenic and chemical nature of the infective agents, the reasons for the phenomena may become apparent.

It has been seen in Chapter 4 that the infectivity of an organism depends upon four things:

(1) Invasiveness
(2) Ability to find suitable tissue in which to live and multiply
(3) Ability to do damage
(4) Communicability

Each of these factors may vary and the infectivity of an organism is the sum total of these attributes. As has been noted, there are some organisms which on some occasions cause diseases which are extremely infectious, and on others cause diseases which are much less infectious because they are confined to a part of the body where they are localized by the body's defences.

The clinical course of an infectious disease is modified considerably by the resistance of the host, so that a haemolytic streptococcus may cause a mild sore throat in one patient and a fulminating scarlet fever in another patient. Both patients are liberating a pathogenic organism from their throats and both are infectious, the difference between the two patients' response is determined by their resistance; the patient with the milder reaction having developed certain protective antibodies including the one to the antigen causing the rash.

It was customary in previous generations to nurse patients suffering from the most infectious diseases in special infectious disease units. The accent, however, should be on the word *most*. All diseases and lesions caused by bacteria, rickettsia, or virus are infectious in that they can be transmitted from one patient to another, either directly or indirectly; the difference is only a matter of degree.

The list of patients with diseases for the treatment of which they are nursed in general wards or infectious disease units respectively, is being gradually revised as more is learnt about the mode of spread and the causative organisms, and about hygiene and therapy. As a rule patients with diseases which are most infectious and which cause serious illnesses are nursed in isolation rooms, are barrier nursed, or are treated in special units.

The position, however, is far from satisfactory. Hospital accommodation is limited and it is sometimes, regrettably, necessary to nurse open cases of tuberculosis (that is to say patients whose sputum contains tubercle bacilli) in general medical wards full of patients whose resistance is lowered by other disease. Patients with multiple staphylococcal lesions, such as boils, or with pneumonia, are nursed in an open ward, and the greatest possible care must be taken if these organisms are not to be disseminated in the bed clothes, by dust and by direct contact. Nursing staff and all who come in contact with patients suffering from an infectious disease must be made aware of the source of infection and relative danger of spread in every case with which they come in contact.

The word contagion is sometimes used to denote the spread of infection by contact either with the infected patient himself or with something he has touched; but provided an infected patient can expel the causative organism in such a manner that it can reach a susceptible host, that host may get the disease. Contagion implies that closer contact with an infected patient is usually necessary to contract the disease; but the word has, however, lost much of its meaning today.

In considering infectious diseases, thought immediately goes to the acute specific fevers like measles and whooping cough which sweep through the community in epidemics, attacking principally the children because the young have developed little or no resistance to the infective agents. The so-called acute specific fevers are a group of diseases caused by bacteria and viruses whose principle difference from the other bacterial and virus diseases is their high degree of infectivity, so that they tend to occur in large outbreaks.

In Chapter 8 and Appendix I the various common pathogenic bacteria, with the diseases which they cause, are described and shown in tabular form. Only those causing disease in temperate climates have been included. It will be seen that one organism may be able to cause lesions in different parts of the body, producing widely different clinical pictures, the infectivity varying with the part attacked and sometimes with the stage of the disease.

Practical Demonstrations

In order to demonstrate the bacterial flora normally present in, for instance, a hospital ward, or on or in the body, it is usual to make cultures of the bacteria on blood agar plates. These plates, when exposed to contamination by the bacteria, are incubated for 18 hours at 37° C and are then examined in a good light. Any colonies should be examined for size, shape, colour, consistency and regularity, and also for any effect on the surrounding red cells in the blood agar. Representatives of each type should be picked off and stained with Gram's stain. The individual and colonial morphology may in some cases be sufficient to identify the organism and, in any case, will indicate what further tests are necessary for complete identification. These tests will include staining and microscopic examination of glass slides, in addition to tests with special media to determine the biochemical activity of organisms, etc.

Preparation of the Slide

To prepare a slide:

1. Clean a slide and place on it one drop of saline.
2. Flame a 1 mm wire loop and cool it.
3. Pick the appropriate colony from the plate with the sterilized loop and emulsify it in the prepared drop of saline. Re-sterilize the loop.
4. Allow the slide to dry.
5. Fix the slide by passing it quickly through the flame. The heat coagulates the proteins in the discharge and the bacteria, fixing them to the glass so that they are not washed off during staining.

Staining the Slide by Gram's Method

For this purpose the solutions in general use are:

(*a*) Methyl violet 6B, 0·5% solution in distilled water.

(*b*) Iodine solution made as follows:

> Iodine 1 g
> Potassium iodide 2 g
> Distilled water to 100 ml

> To counterstain use:

(*c*) Neutral red solution, made as follows:

> Neutral red 1 g
> 1% acetic acid 2 ml
> Distilled water to 1000 ml

Technique

1. Methyl violet solution is poured over the whole slide and left for 30 seconds.
2. Excess stain is poured off, and what remains of it is washed off with iodine solution, which is left on for 1 minute.
3. The iodine solution is washed off with alcohol, and such washing is continued until no more colour is removed from the preparation.
4. The preparation is next washed with water.
5. The slide is flooded with counterstain and left for 2 minutes.
6. The slide is once more washed with water and dried between layers of blotting paper.

The slide may then be examined under the oil-immersion lens of a microscope.

Demonstrations of Ward Bacterial Flora

Demonstration 1

Expose blood agar plates for half an hour in the following places:

  (i) Near an open door.
 (ii) On a window sill.
(iii) In the middle of the ward before and after bed-making.
(iv) Beside a bed during bedmaking with a minimum disturbance of blankets.
 (v) Beside a bed during bedmaking with a maximum disturbance of blankets.

Expected Results. On exposures (i), (ii) and (iii) the following organisms may be found:

    (*a*) Aerobic spore-bearing bacilli
    (*b*) Non-pathogenic staphylococci
    (*c*) Non-haemolytic streptococci
    (*d*) Micrococci
    (*e*) Diphtheroids

On exposures (iv) and (v), the above-mentioned organisms are likely to be found with, in addition, the following:

    (*f*) Pathogenic staphylococci
    (*g*) Coliform organisms
    (*h*) Haemolytic and other forms of streptococci

The bacterial flora of a ward will vary with the time of day at which the plates are exposed, the weather, the type of room and its position, but it is to be expected that there will be more colonies on those plates which have been exposed in places where there is a draught of air. Plate counts will be higher, therefore, by the door, on a window sill and near a bed that is being made than in the centre of the ward where the air is relatively still.

Demonstration 2

Inoculate swabs taken from the following places on to blood agar plates:

  (i) Grease marks round the bath and basin after use.

  (ii) Surface of prepared sterile dressing trolley before use.

  (iii) Surface of prepared sterile dressing trolley after use.

  (iv) Racks where bedpans are kept.

  (v) Ward blankets.

Expected Results. (i) The organisms found may be of types *a* to *e* in the above list.

(ii) A correctly prepared trolley shows no bacterial growth before use.

(iii) A dressing trolley after use may show organisms of types *a* to *e* inclusive and also others depending upon the type of dressing for which the trolley was used.

(iv) Organisms of types *a*, *b*, *c*, and *g* are likely to be found on swabs from bedpan racks.

(v) Blankets and bedclothes contain very many mixed organisms, the type depending upon the predominating flora in the immediate vicinity and those carried by the occupant of the bed. Disturbance of the bedclothes during making of beds causes many of these to be shaken from the blankets and into the air; this will be apparent when the plates which have been exposed during bedmaking are examined.

Demonstration of the Normal Flora from Available Body Surfaces

Demonstration 1

(i) Place the fingers on the surface of a blood agar plate.

(ii) Wash hands in soapy water, scrub nails with a soft brush, rinse under running water and place the fingers on the surface of a blood agar plate.

(iii) Comb the hair over a blood agar plate.

(iv) Take a throat swab, inoculate on blood agar plates by rubbing the swab gently on the surface.

(v) Take duplicate nose and ear swabs, and (*a*) inoculate one pair on to blood agar plates directly, (*b*) place the other pair into their appropriate tubes containing disinfectant, e.g. Roccal 1 in 40, and leave for half an hour. Then inoculate swabs on blood agar plates.

(vi) Sneeze over a blood agar plate and cough over another.

Expected Results. (i) Organisms of types *a*, *b*, and *c* are normally found on the skin, while pathogenic staphylococci (type *f*) are frequently found on normal fingers.

(ii) The bacterial count will be reduced by washing but the hands are not necessarily made bacteria-free. Sometimes they appear to be increased in number (p. 76).

(iii) Organisms of types *a*, *b*, *c* and *f* are frequently found on plates over which hair has been combed.

(iv) On throat swabs any of the following may be found:

Non-pathogenic staphylococci.
Non-haemolytic and *viridans* type streptococci (those which cause a green coloration round the colonies growing on a blood agar plate).
Non-pathogenic haemolytic streptococci (those which produce a clear halo round the colonies when growing on a blood agar plate). It is important to note that not all haemolytic streptococci are pathogenic— further tests must be applied to pick out those which are harmful.

> Diphtheroids
> Micrococci
> Pneumococci
> Non-pathogenic neisseriae
> *Haemophilus influenzae*

(v) On nose and ear swabs may be found organisms of types *a*, *b*, and *c*.

It is important to remember that vessels for taking specimens should be sterile, that is to say free from organisms, but should contain no disinfectant or agent which may kill any organisms that may be put in with the specimen.

Demonstrations to Test the Efficiency of Sterilization Technique

In order to test the efficiency of sterilization by the autoclave, a number of tests may be applied:

Demonstration 1

A box of theatre towels, folded and rolled correctly, is packed so that there is room for the free penetration of steam. In the centre of the box are placed:

(i) A piece of fusible metal which melts at 120° C in a bijou bottle.

(ii) A piece of string impregnated with spores of *Bacillus subtilis* in a bijou bottle, either loosely plugged with wool or with the cap half screwed up.

The box is then sent to be sterilized in the usual manner with the ventilators open if drums are used.

Expected Results. The metal will have melted and there will be no bacterial growth. Sterilization will have been adequate.

Demonstration 2

The procedure outlined for demonstration above is repeated, the box this time being sent for sterilization with the ventilators shut, so that the steam cannot penetrate.

Expected Results. There will be bacterial growth but the metal may have melted; that is to say the required temperature may have been reached in the centre of the box, but closed ventilators will have prevented the steam from penetrating and sterilization will not have been achieved.

Demonstration 3

A box of theatre towels is packed folded but not rolled. These are placed in the box as tightly as possible, the fusible metal and spore string being included, and the box sent for sterilization.

The following points are noted:

(c) Whether the metal has melted;
(b) Whether growth occurs on the string impregnated with *Bacillus subtilis* after broth has been poured on to it and it has been incubated at 37° C for 18 hours.

Expected Results. In this instance also the metal may have melted, but there may be bacterial growth because tight packing has prevented free penetration of the steam. Melting of the metal indicates only that the stated temperature has been reached; it gives no indication of how long this temperature was maintained.

Demonstration 4

A piece of gauze swab is impregnated with a broth culture of:

(i) Staphylococci,
(ii) *Bacillus subtilis*, a spore-producing, non-pathogenic organism.

Each swab is placed in a separate, covered enamel dish and boiled for 5 minutes. Each piece of gauze is taken from the dishes with sterile forceps and dropped into a tube of broth. The broths are incubated for 18 hours at 37° C, and note is made of any growth.

Expected Results. There will be no bacterial growth

from the swab impregnated with staphylococci; 5 minutes' boiling is sufficient to kill many non-spore-bearing organisms. There will be growth from the swab impregnated with *B. subtilis*; 5 minutes' boiling is insufficient to kill the spore-bearing organisms if these, at the time of the test, are in the spore-bearing form. The only sure method of killing spores is autoclaving.

7 NORMAL FLORA OF THE HUMAN BODY

NURSES do not need to have much detailed knowledge of microorganisms, but some notes on the normal flora present on the skin and other body surfaces and on the commoner pathogenic organisms are included in this book for purposes of reference. The material is also presented shortly in tabular form, stressing the practical points of the route of entry and exit in each disease so that the nurse can deal with each patient intelligently, and readily avoid the spread of infection to other persons and to herself (Chapter 11).

All areas of the body in contact with the atmosphere can harbour bacteria, so that it is the rule to find organisms on the skin and the mucous membranes of the respiratory tract, the alimentary canal and the vagina; it is neither normal nor desirable to have no bacteria on these sites. Organisms living a harmless existence in these sites are non-pathogenic and are considered the normal flora of the part. Should they, however, leave that site and lodge in another site, they may cause damage. *Escherichia coli* (*Bacterium coli*), for instance, is a normal inhabitant of the intestinal tract; such bacteria do not cause damage and do not invade. If, however, they enter the urethra the same organisms may produce an infection of the urinary tract.

Thus some organisms which occur as normal flora in the human body are non-pathogenic; others are non-pathogenic in their usual site, probably due to their inability to get through the particular surface which is their normal habitat and invade the tissues, but they may be pathogenic in another site.

In certain conditions the surfaces normally harbouring a mixed flora of non-pathogenic organisms may become damaged or blocked, allowing organisms usually considered of low-grade pathogenicity to invade the damaged mucosa and cause disease. This is well seen in various bronchitic and bronchiectatic conditions. Damage to the bronchial mucosa by a virus infection or by smoking sometimes results in a febrile condition with the production of much sputum. Microbiological investigation of this sputum reveals only organisms which are considered normal respiratory tract flora and which under normal conditions do not cause lesions in the respiratory tract.

Hand-washing before carrying out preparations for surgical dressings, etc., is designed to remove recently acquired bacteria which might easily become detached and contaminate objects at this stage. However, it is also important to remember that sweat on a clean, healthy skin has antiseptic properties; indeed, it has been demonstrated that more organisms grow on recently washed skin than on clean skin not recently washed. This obviously has some bearing on routine hand-washing and the preparation of skin for injections, but the final conclusions to be drawn from trials conducted to test the validity of observations such as these have not yet been reached. Another fact to note is that, as has already been mentioned, hydrochloric acid and bile keep the multiplication of intestinal flora in check. The thoughtful nurse should keep all these complex points in mind.

8 A GUIDE TO COMMON PATHOGENIC ORGANISMS

How to Understand Laboratory Reports

WHEN writing a report the medical microbiologist has two tasks, namely, the giving of factual information for the hospital records, and comment on the facts when this seems necessary. It is not necessary for the microbiologist to comment on every organism found in certain specimens, for doctors know the names of common organisms, their relative powers of producing disease, and in general their significance in the material.

Let us look at the kind of report which may be sent out several times a day from any busy laboratory:

Request:
> Pus from abscess, opened in axilla, for organisms.

Report:
> Swab bearing *thick pus*.
>
> Direct smear showed pus cells and clusters of Gram positive cocci.
>
> Culture yielded a *coagulase-positive staphylococcus*, sensitive to tetracycline but insensitive to penicillin.

This report first describes the material received and secondly its appearance when stained to show organisms under the microscope, though without naming the microorganisms. The third statement names the microorganisms in a special way so that the doctor reading the report will know immediately that the staphylococcus is the causal organism in this instance. The important words in the report are underlined. In itself the presence of pus indicates inflammation, and such material is the best source of a causal organism. The fact that the staphylococcus produced the substance coagulase implies that this particular organism was pathogenic (p. 86). To know this fact, of course, is to have specialized knowledge, and all doctors must have a minimum amount of such knowledge. It is important for either a doctor or a nurse to know that only pathogenic staphylococci produce this substance coagulase. It is not so important for a nurse to know any other facts about staphylococci unless she wishes to do so, although it will help her understanding of disease mechanisms if she knows a little about the microorganisms. The aim in this chapter is to present some outstanding facts about common organisms which the nurse may use for quick reference when she meets them in laboratory reports.

The Main Divisions of Microorganisms

The population of the microbiological world can be grouped into six divisions:

  I Non-branching organisms stained by crystal violet + iodine (Gram positive)
 II Non-branching organisms not stained by crystal violet + iodine (Gram negative)
III Branching organisms, Gram positive and Gram negative
IV Organisms stained by hot basic fuchsin (acid-fast)
 V Organisms not stained by the above dyes (spirochaetes)
VI Organisms only seen inside stained cells (viruses)

Most of the organisms have two or even three names, and in the pages that follow the present international name used by microbiologists is given first, followed by the common names used in Britain before the international nomenclature was adopted.

I GRAM POSITIVE DIVISION

(1) CORYNEBACTERIUM

Thick skinned rod. Found on skin and mucous membranes.

PATHOGENIC	HARMLESS
C. diphtheriae, or diphtheria bacillus, or Klebs-Loeffler bacillus. Usual portal of entry is the upper respiratory tract, but occasionally the vagina, the skin or the conjunctiva. Spread by human carriers. Cause of **diphtheria.**	*C. hofmannii, C. xerosis*

C. diphtheriae is distinguished from the harmless members of the group by biochemical tests, but principally by toxin-production, which is shown by injecting cultures of the organism into the skin of the guinea pig; a red patch appears after two to four days. The Schick test is an intradermal test with toxin which determines a patient's susceptibility to diphtheria.

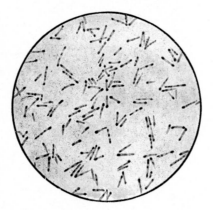

FIG. 20

Corynebacterium diphtheriae, OR DIPHTHERIA BACILLUS.

(2) BACILLUS

Rod with spores, aerobe. Found in air, soil, water, dust, wool, hair, carcases.

PATHOGENIC

B. anthracis, or anthrax bacillus. Enters through the skin, or spores inhaled into the lungs pass into the blood stream. Spread by animals and animal products, such as hides, hair, wool, infected carcases and bedding. Cause of **anthrax.**

HARMLESS

B. subtilis. Often used as test organism for checking effectiveness of sterilization procedures. Spores dried on string are put into test bottles for packing into drums, boxes or packs.

B. anthracis is distinguished from the harmless members of the group by biochemical tests and pathogenicity tests in animals.

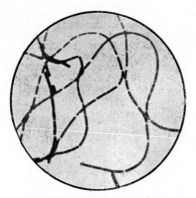

Fig. 21.—*Bacillus anthracis* FROM AGAR CULTURE
($\times$ 750).

(3)   CLOSTRIDIUM

Rod with spore, shaped like spindle, key or tennis racket. Found everywhere in air, soil, excreta and all kinds of putrefying material. Many members are harmless (*Cl. sporogenes*) and even the pathogenic members may not cause disease unless the spores are carried into wounds, or material where conditions are exactly suitable for growth and toxin production.

PATHOGENIC MEMBERS

Cl. tetani, or Bacillus tetani. Produces toxin when carried into wounds. This poisons motor nerves, with an effect not unlike strychnine, resulting in the disease **tetanus.**	*Cl. perfringens* (or *welchii*), or *Bacillus welchii.* Produces toxin when carried into wounds or limbs with damaged blood supply. The muscular damage produced is known as **gas gangrene.** Other gas gangrene producers are *Cl. septique* and *Cl. oedematiens.*	*Cl. botulinum,* or *Bacillus botulinum.* Produces toxin in tinned, potted or semi-cooked food. The poisoned food when eaten causes acute toxaemia characterized by paralysis of the cranial motor nerves and of the diaphragm which is known as **botulism.**

Certain strains of *Cl. perfringens* are associated with a mild form of food poisoning (pp. 122, 172).

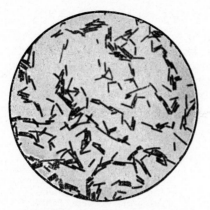

FIG. 22.—*Clostridium perfringens*, OR *Bacillus welchii*, FROM AGAR CULTURE (× 800).

The cause of gas gangrene.

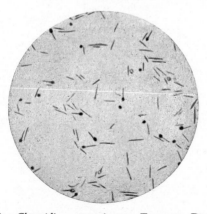

FIG. 23.—*Clostridium tetani*, OR TETANUS BACILLUS, FROM AGAR CULTURE (× 800).

The cause of tetanus.

(4) STREPTOCOCCUS

Egg-shaped or rounded bodies in pairs or chains like strings of beads. Found everywhere. Many inhabit mucous membranes of man and animals, including mouth, upper respiratory tract and intestine. Many live in food, especially milk and dairy products, where they are found with the *lactobacillus*. Some kinds discolour or destroy red blood cells and are called 'haemolytic streptococci'.

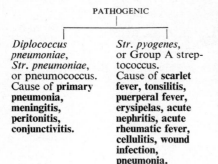

PATHOGENIC

Diplococcus pneumoniae, *Str. pneumoniae,* or pneumococcus. Cause of **primary pneumonia, meningitis, peritonitis, conjunctivitis.**

Str. pyogenes, or Group A streptococcus. Cause of **scarlet fever, tonsilitis, puerperal fever, erysipelas, acute nephritis, acute rheumatic fever, cellulitis, wound infection, pneumonia.**

HARMLESS TO MAN—many hundreds of strains—except streptococci of the *viridans* group and closely related organisms which may cause **subacute bacterial endocarditis.**

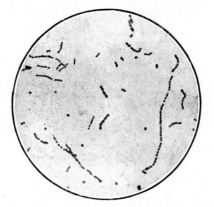

FIG. 24.—*Streptococcus pyogenes*, OR GROUP A
STREPTOCOCCUS, FROM BROTH CULTURE (× 950).

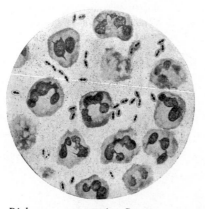

FIG. 25.—*Diplococcus pneumoniae, Streptococcus pneumoniae*,
OR PNEUMOCOCCI, IN FILM OF PUS, STAINED TO SHOW CAPSULES
(× 950).

(5) STAPHYLOCOCCUS

Balls in clusters like grapes. Found in air, soil, on mucous membranes and skin.

PATHOGENIC	HARMLESS
Staphylococcus aureus, or *coagulase-positive staphylococcus*, sometimes called *Staph. pyogenes*. Usually enters through the skin, but may enter through mucous membranes. Spread by human carriers and found in about 50% of people, especially in hospital staff. Cause of all kinds of **abscesses, boils, carbuncles, whitlows, styes, breast abscess, pemphigus neonatorum, infected wounds, secondary infection of lung in influenzal pneumonia, and in food poisoning.**	Coagulase-negative, found in nose and on the skin.

The principal organisms causing food poisoning are mentioned on pp. 82 and 94. The spread of staphylococcal infection is shown in the illustrations on pp. 21 and 25.

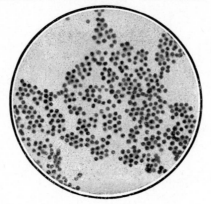

Fig. 26.

Staphylococcus aureus FROM AGAR CULTURE (× 950).

Streptococci and Staphylococci

Grouping of streptococci is done by a special chemical test in which part of the bacterial protoplasm is extracted and mixed with various antisera. There are at least 13 groups labelled from A to O, and 90% of streptococci from human infections belong to Group A, which is the important group for the nurse to remember. Occasionally human infections are caused by strains belonging to Group C or Group G, and that is why reports state whether a haemolytic streptococcus does or does not belong to one of these Groups A, C or G. During an outbreak of streptococcal infection in hospital wards or schools, it may be necessary to distinguish between two or more Group A strains. This is done by serological tests which distinguish between about 40 different types. The spread of streptococcal infection is illustrated on pp. 20 and 25.

Typing of coagulase-positive staphylococci plays an important part in the controlling of cross-infection in hospital wards. There are 20 or more *types* of staphylococcus and the bacteriologist tries to find out which particular type is the cause of cross-infection at one time. General swabbings are carried out on staff and patients to find the troublesome strain and to try to trace its spread from person to person. Sometimes the source may be the nose of the individual whose wound becomes infected, an example of bacteria which are saprophytic in one situation and pathogenic in another. This is 'auto-infection'.

II   GRAM NEGATIVE DIVISION

(1) NEISSERIA

Bean-shaped bodies in pairs, often seen inside pus cells. Found on mucous membranes, particularly upper respiratory tract, genito-urinary tract and conjunctiva.

PATHOGENIC		HARMLESS
N. gonorrhoeae, or gonococcus. Enters through mucous membrane of genito-urinary tract or conjunctiva. Cause of **gonorrhoea** and of some cases of purulent ophthalmia. Usually seen in direct smears of pus from urethritis and cervicitis and grown in cultures of pus made at the bedside or in the clinic.	*N. meningitidis*, or meningococcus. Enters through mucous membrane of upper respiratory tract, thence to blood stream and central nervous system. Cause of **cerebro-spinal fever.** Also called meningo-coccal meningitis. Found in cerebro-spinal fluid in cases of meningitis and usually easily seen in direct smears.	*N. catarrhalis*, often reported in sputum.

Both these pathogenic organisms die very quickly outside the body and this must be remembered when material for culture is being taken.

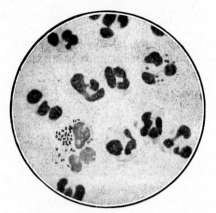

FIG. 27.—*Neisseria gonorrhoeae*, OR GONOCOCCI, IN PUS
(× 950).

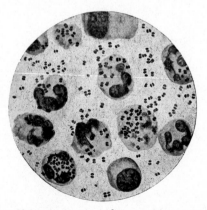

FIG. 28.—*Neisseria meningitidis*, OR MENINGOCOCCI, IN
PURULENT CEREBROSPINAL FLUID.

(2) HAEMOPHILUS

Very small organisms, usually rods, but may be almost any shape. Usually inhabit mucous membranes of man and animals.

PATHOGENIC   HARMLESS

Strains of *H. influenzae* found in nasal sinuses and sputum of older children and adults.

H. ducreyi. Enters by mucous membrane of genital tract. Cause of **soft sore** or soft chancre.

*H. influenzae,** or Pfeiffer's bacillus. Certain pathogenic strains enter through upper respiratory tract and pass via blood stream into central nervous system of infants. May also enter through conjunctiva. Cause of **infantile meningitis** and **conjunctivitis.** Often found in patients with chronic bronchitis.

*Once thought to be the cause of influenza, which we now know is caused by a virus.

Bordetella pertussis, *H. pertussis,* or Bordet-Gengou bacillus. Enters by upper respiratory tract. Cause of **whooping cough** or **pertussis.**

(3) BRUCELLA

Very small rods. Inhabit animals, particularly cattle, sheep, goats and swine, and live in milk of cattle and goats. All the brucellae seem to be pathogenic for man.

Br. suis.
Found in swine.
Cause of a type of **undulant fever.**
Common in the U.S. but not in Great Britain.

Br. abortus.
Found in cattle.
Cause of **undulant fever** or abortus fever. Cause of **abortion in cattle** in Great Britain.

Br. melitensis.
Found in goats.
Cause of **undulant fever** or Malta fever. Common in Mediterranean countries but not in Great Britain.

All the brucellae enter through the mucous membranes of the intestine, either by infected milk or indirectly through personal contact with infected animals. In Great Britain the disease is generally spread through batches of infected milk, though brucellosis is still fairly common in farm hands and veterinary workers. From the intestine the organisms pass into the blood stream, and may be grown from samples of the patient's blood (blood culture). Patients may develop antibodies detectable in serum agglutinin tests, and these tests are carried out on sera of patients with pyrexia of unknown origin.

(4) PASTEURELLA

Very small rods with polar granules. Inhabit insects, particularly fleas and ticks, which pass them on to rodents, which in turn infect other insects. Human beings may become involved in the pasteurellae life cycle if brought in contact with certain insects and certain rodents. Some of the pasteurellae are found in animals, (e.g. cats) without any known intervention by insects.

Fransicella tularensis.* P. pestis.
Inhabits ticks which bite rats and squirrels, which infect other ticks which bite men, causing **tularaemia.** Unknown in Great Britain, well known in the United States.

P. pestis.
Inhabits the rat flea, which lives on blood of the two plague rats. Other fleas bite the infected rats and then bite men, causing **bubonic** or **pneumonic plague.**

P. septica.**
Carried by domestic cats which transfer the organism by a bite or scratch causing **abscess** and **septicaemia.**

This is not the cause of **cat scratch fever, which is caused by a virus.

* Formerly called *Pasteurella*

In all these infections the organisms usually enter by puncture of the skin, thence via lymphatics to blood stream but they may also be inhaled. This latter is the mode of infection in pneumonic plague. Tularaemia is generally acquired by persons who handle infected animal carcases.

(5) ENTEROBACTERIACEAE

Small rods, sometimes motile, sometimes capsulated. Widely distributed in nature, especially in fresh water, and able to live independently. Some members inhabit the human intestines, the genitalia and the respiratory tract. Some are pathogenic and in the faeces, for example, coliform group bacteria are 'normal flora'.

(i) Escherichia and Klebsiella

Escherichia coli, or *Bacterium coli,* or *Bacillus coli.*

Klebsiella aerogenes or *Aerobacter aerogenes.*

Klebsiella pneumoniae, or *Bacterium friedländeri,* or *Friedländer's bacillus.*

Found in urinary tract in pyelitis, pyelonephritis and cystitis. Also found in wounds and may occasionally cause meningitis. Certain types of *E. coli* are associated with neonatal gastroenteritis.

Found in respiratory tract and responsible for about 3% of cases of pneumonia.

These organisms are distinguished from each other by biochemical tests.

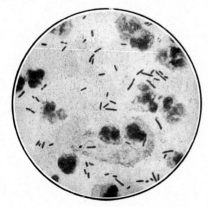

FIG. 29.—*Escherichia coli*, OR *Bacterium coli*, IN DEPOSIT OF URINE FROM CASE OF CYSTITIS (× 950).

(ii) Salmonella

Small rod, indistinguishable from *bacterium* except by biochemical and serological tests, and inhabits the same places. All members are potentially pathogenic.

ENTERIC FEVER
GROUP

FOOD POISONING
GROUP

More than 800 types, named after places all over the world, *e.g. Salm. montevideo.*

Common in Great Britain. *Salm. typhimurium, Salm. enteritidis.* Enter intestine in food, not usually carried into blood stream.

Salm. paratyphi B. Cause of para-typhoid fever in Great Britain. *Salm. paratyphi A.* Common in Asia. *Salm. paratyphi C.* Uncommon in Great Britain, common in Europe.

Salm. typhi, or *Bacillus typhosus,* or *Bacterium typhosum.* Cause of **typhoid.**

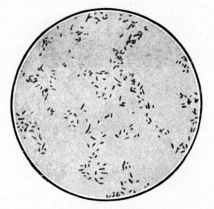

Fig. 30.—*Salmonella typhi*, or Typhoid Bacillus, from Agar Culture.

Salm. typhi enters intestine by contaminated food, milk, water or direct contact of contaminated articles, passes into lymphatics, thence to blood stream and bone marrow, and back to lymphoid tissue of reticulo-endothelial system. It is excreted in faeces and urine but may also be passed from the mouth by some patients.

(iii) Shigella

Small rod, indistinguishable from *bacterium*, but non-motile. Found in the same places as *bacteria*, but potentially pathogenic for susceptible people.

Sh. shiga.	*Sh. flexneri.*	*Sh. sonnei.*	*Sh. boydii.*
Very rare in Great Britain.	6 types, fairly common in Great Britain.	Very common in Great Britain.	Several types, rare in Great Britain.

The organisms are the cause of **bacterial dysentery.** They are distinguished from bacteria and salmonellae by biochemical and serological tests. Infection is spread by human carriers (p. 25). The organisms enter the mucous membrane of the large intestine. Besides those mentioned above, *Sh. schmitzi, Sh. alkalescens* and *Sh. dispar* are occasionally found in Great Britain. *Sh. sonnei* is usually found in children, and *Sh. flexneri* is common among patients in mental institutions.

(6) PROTEUS, PSEUDOMONAS AND VIBRIO

Motile rods which are self-sufficient and independent, inhabiting air, soil and water, and found in excreta of man and animals. *Proteus* and *Pseudomonas* are secondary invaders when some other organism has caused the primary infection.

Proteus is also a member of the family of the enterobacteriaceae, but *pseudomonas* and *vibrio* are not. There are now four species of *Proteus*, but the one most often found in human infections is *P. mirabilis*.

RELATIVELY HARMFUL

PATHOGENIC

Proteus mirabilis or *Bacillus proteus*. Found in urinary infections and wounds. Causes smell of 'bad fish'.

Pseudomonas aeruginosa, *Pseudomonas pyocyanea*, or *Bacillus pyocyaneus*. Found in urinary infections and wounds. Causes **blue pus.**

Vibrio cholerae, or Comma bacillus. Cause of **Asiatic cholera.**

III BRANCHING BACTERIA AND ACTINOMYCETACEAE

A huge family of organisms which may be Gram positive, Gram negative or intermediate. They are distinguished from other bacteria because they form branches and grow into microscopic trees or bushes (mycelium). They inhabit soil, air, plants and animals, and include the streptomyces (source of streptomycin and other antibiotics).

GRAM POSITIVE MEMBERS

(1) Club-ended rods, bush-like growth

Anaerobes	Aerobes	
Actinomyces israeli. Method of entry variable. Causes chronic granular lesions of bones, lungs, caecum and appendix, known as **actinomycosis.**	*Nocardia madurae.* Cause of the tropical disease **Madura foot.**	*Nocardia aster-oides.* Causes of **chronic abscess in lungs and muscles.**

(2) Rudimentary branching, straggling growth

Erysipelothrix rhusiopathiae, or swine fever bacillus. Enters through scratch or skin puncture by some article infected by rats or by infected swine. Causes cellulitis of hand and forearm called **erysipeloid** seen often in fish porters. When caught from infected swine there is usually a fatal septicaemia.	*Actinomyces muris,* or *Streptobaccillus moniliformis.* Enters through skin by rat bite or scratch, but may be taken in infected milk. Causes fever, rash, endocarditis and polyarthritis, which is sometimes called **Haverhill fever or rat-bite fever.**

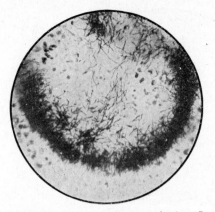

FIG. 31.—COLONY OF *Actinomyces bovis* IN LIVER
(× 800).

GRAM NEGATIVE MEMBERS

(1) Fusiform or spindle-like anaerobes

Fusiformis necroforus.
Found in intestine, in **appendix abscess,** in necrotic skin lesions, such as the **dry gangrene of diabetes.**
Already present in body and ready to take advantage of anaerobic conditions.

*Fusiformis vincentii,** or fusiform bacillus.

* *F. vincentii,* accompanied by *Borrelia vincentii* (pp. 102, 176.), is found in smears of mouth, gums and fauces in the **ulcerative gingivitis** known as **Vincent's angina.**

(2) *Mycoplasma.*
Many shapes and sizes, aerobes, difficult to grow.
Group also known as PPLO or pleuro-pneu-monia-like organisms, so called because they resemble the organisms which cause pleuro-pneumonia of cattle. Found on mucous membranes of eyes and genitalia.
M. pneumoniae causes **primary atypical pneumonia.**

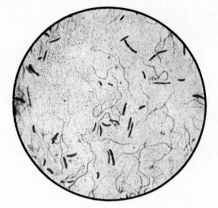

FIG. 32.
SPIROCHAETES AND
FUSIFORM BACILLI
FROM THROAT OF A
CASE OF VINCENT'S
ANGINA (× 950).

IV ACID-FAST DIVISION

MYCOBACTERIUM

Slender rods, granular (like the corynebacteria), which may show rudimentary branching, and are enveloped win unsaponifiable wax which renders the organisms difficult to stain by Gram's method. After staining by hot carbol fuchsin, the organisms are stain-fast, resisting decolorization with alcohols and strong mineral acids.

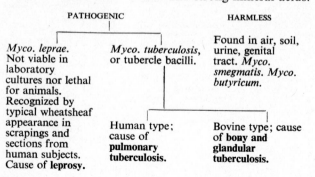

PATHOGENIC		HARMLESS
Myco. leprae. Not viable in laboratory cultures nor lethal for animals. Recognized by typical wheatsheaf appearance in scrapings and sections from human subjects. Cause of **leprosy.**	*Myco. tuberculosis,* or tubercle bacilli.	Found in air, soil, urine, genital tract. *Myco. smegmatis. Myco. butyricum.*
	Human type; cause of **pulmonary tuberculosis.**	Bovine type; cause of **bony and glandular tuberculosis.**

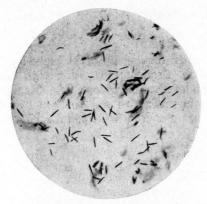

FIG. 33.—*Mycobacterium tuberculosis*, OR TUBERCLE BACILLI, FROM CULTURE (× 800).

Myco. tuberculosis is a slow-growing organism, and though the organism may be seen in direct smears, no growth may appear in cultures for several weeks. Even in a susceptible animal like the guinea pig typical lesions may not develop for several weeks, therefore the diagnosis of tuberculosis in the absence of positive direct smears may necessarily be delayed.

V 'UNSTAINABLE' DIVISION

SPIROCHAETES

Slender rods, moving by rapid snake-like and corkscrew motion. Brought into vision with dark ground illumination of the microscope field because they are difficult or impossible to stain by usual methods. The organisms are grown in tissue cultures containing living cells.

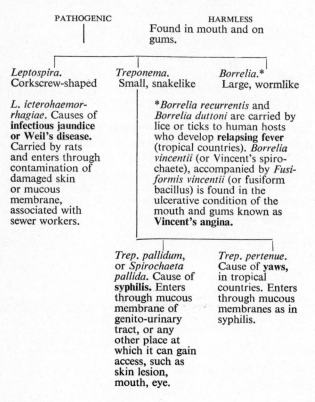

PATHOGENIC

HARMLESS
Found in mouth and on gums.

Leptospira.
Corkscrew-shaped

Treponema.
Small, snakelike

*Borrelia.**
Large, wormlike

L. icterohaemor-rhagiae. Causes of **infectious jaundice or Weil's disease.** Carried by rats and enters through contamination of damaged skin or mucous membrane, associated with sewer workers.

Borrelia recurrentis* and *Borrelia duttoni* are carried by lice or ticks to human hosts who develop **relapsing fever (tropical countries). *Borrelia vincentii* (or Vincent's spirochaete), accompanied by *Fusiformis vincentii* (or fusiform bacillus) is found in the ulcerative condition of the mouth and gums known as **Vincent's angina.**

Trep. pallidum, or *Spirochaeta pallida.* Cause of **syphilis.** Enters through mucous membrane of genito-urinary tract, or any other place at which it can gain access, such as skin lesion, mouth, eye.

Trep. pertenue. Cause of **yaws,** in tropical countries. Enters through mucous membranes as in syphilis.

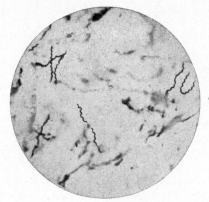

FIG. 34.
Treponema pallidum,
OR *Spirochaeta pallida,*
IN LYMPH GLAND.
WARTHIN'S STAIN
(× 800).

VI RICKETTSIA

Rickettsiae are intermediate between bacteria and viruses. They grow only in susceptible tissue cells of certain animals, and in nature are carried by many different kinds of insects.

R. prowazeki.
Cause of **epidemic typhus,** is carried by lice.

R. orientalis.
Cause of **scrub typhus,** is carried by mites.

R. rickettsi.
Cause of **spotted fever,** is carried by ticks.

Each of the different forms of typhus and spotted fever is caused by different rickettsiae, which are carried by insects indigenous to the places where they occur, e.g. Rocky Mountain spotted fever, South African tick-bite fever, Queensland tick-bite fever. Q fever caused by *R. burnetii* has occurred in Britain since the Second World War.

VII VIRUSES

The many varieties of virus and the diseases that they cause are dealt with in Chapter 9.

9 COMMON VIRAL DISEASES

VIRUSES are particles so small that many of them are invisible with the light microscope, though they have been studied with the electron microscope. Clumps of virus particles may sometimes be seen in tissue cells, when they form part of structures known as inclusion bodies. Neither viruses nor rickettsiae (p. 9) can grow on lifeless culture media, but only in the living cells of man and other animals which are susceptible to infection. Besides the many infections which we know to be due to viruses, there are numbers which we believe are due to viruses, because they are undoubtedly infectious and no bacterial cause has been found. Many viruses have been discovered during the last ten years and, with the great advances that have recently been made in technical methods, no doubt many more will be discovered.

Laboratory diagnosis. The isolation and identification of viruses is often a long and complex procedure. After special preparation, clinical materials are inoculated on to tissue cultures or fertile eggs or into susceptible animals, or possibly all three methods may be used. According to their kind, viruses may be isolated from various sources such as pustules or herpetic blisters, throat washings, faeces and rectal swabs, and blood cultures. It is not necessarily of the first importance always to isolate the virus, and it is often easier and quicker to show an immune reaction (p. 59) in the patient's serum than to isolate the virus.

Virus antibodies. Patients produce antibodies to

104

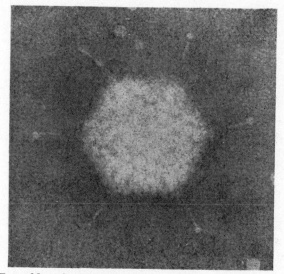

FIG. 35a.—AN ADENOVIRUS AS SEEN THROUGH THE
ELECTRON MICROSCOPE.

viruses, just as they do to bacteria. Many patients may already have antibodies against the commoner viruses left over from a previous infection. If the strength of antibody in the patient's serum changes from one occasion to the next, we may assume that there has probably been a recent infection. It is therefore important to obtain two blood samples from the patient, preferably in the early and last stages of the illnesses, and to compare the strength of the antibody in the two samples. The majority of the viral infections mentioned in the following section can be diagnosed by obtaining serological evidence of infection in this way.

Viruses are divided into groups depending partly on their size, partly on their habitat, partly on the kind of disease produced and partly on some special character-

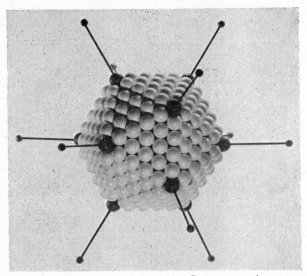

FIG. 35b.—MODEL OF AN ADENOVIRUS SHOWING ITS ANTENNAE.

istic such as the property of sticking on to red blood cells. To get some idea of their size, we can compare them with the size of a staphylococcus, which is $\frac{1}{1000}$ mm or 1 μ across. They vary in size from about one half to one thirtieth the size of the staphylococcus: the sizes of the different types that have been isolated are given as they are dealt with in this chapter.

The Psittacosis-LGV Group

It is now believed that this group of organisms is nearer to the bacteria than to the viruses. A new name has been suggested for them, *Bedsonia*, but has not yet been generally adopted. The methods for their isolation and identification are like those for viruses so it is appropriate to consider them here.

They are relatively large, being about one-third to a half of the size of a staphylococcus. Many of them inhabit birds.

Psittacosis virus causes a pneumonia-like illness, which is sometimes fatal. It is acquired by contact with parrots and budgerigars.

Trachoma virus causes a chronic form of conjunctivitis endemic in North Africa, which may result in blindness.

Lymphogranuloma venereum causes a venereal disease common in the tropics. In the United Kingdom, it is most often seen in seamen and immigrants.

Although these viruses are closely related to each other, each one causes a quite different kind of illness from the others. The diseases all respond to some extent to treatment with the tetracycline drugs, chlortetracycline (Aureomycin), oxytetracycline (Terryamycin) and tetracycline (Achromycin).

The Pox Viruses

The pox viruses are all somewhat rectangular particles about one third to a quarter of the size of a staphylococcus. They inhabit human beings and are transmitted from person to person, causing a generalized disease with characteristically distributed spots.

Variola virus causes smallpox.

Vaccinia virus causes cowpox.

Smallpox vaccination. The two viruses variola and vaccinia are closely related and an attack of cowpox will protect an individual against smallpox for several years. This is the basis for immunization against smallpox by inoculation with vaccinia virus prepared from lesions in calves.

Varicella virus causes chickenpox, but it is also the

cause of herpes zoster (or shingles). A person in contact with a patient with chickenpox may develop shingles, and therefore shingles must be treated with the same care to prevent cross-infection as is chickenpox. Second attacks of both infections are fairly common.

The Myxoviruses

The myxoviruses are spherical and about one-tenth of the size of a staphylococcus. They are able to stick on to human red blood cells causing them to clump together (haemagglutination).

Influenza virus causes epidemic and sporadic cases of influenza. There are three types, known as A, B and C. The cause of the so-called Asian flu is a variant of Type A. One of the most serious complications of influenza is a secondary bacterial infection resulting in pneumonia. The bacteria concerned may be either pathogenic staphylococci, streptococci or *Haemophilus*, and sometimes mixtures of these organisms. *Haemophilus influenzae* acquired its name because of its association with the influenza virus in the great epidemic of 1918.

Mumps virus causes the acute infectious disease of that name, characterized most often by swelling of the parotid glands, though other glandular organs may be affected, for example the pancreas, ovaries and testes.

Both mumps and influenza viruses may cause meningitis (pp. 84, 88).

The Arboviruses

The arboviruses are about one twenty-fifth of the size of a staphylococcus. Arbo is a shortened form of 'arthropod-borne' meaning 'carried by insects' such as mosquitoes. They are also known as 'arbo viruses'. The viruses are transmitted to human beings by insect bites.

Subgroup (*1*) contains twelve viruses all of which cause encephalitis. Each virus has its own geographical distribution. Some examples are St Louis encephalitis virus, Japanese B virus and Russian spring–summer fever virus, which are all transmitted by mosquito bites.

Subgroup (*2*) contains several viruses all causing a generalized febrile disease. Each virus also has its own geographical distribution. Some examples are *yellow fever, dengue, sand-fly fever* and *Rift Valley fever*. There is a yellow fever vaccine which has been used effectively to immunize people entering the yellow fever zones. Obviously another method of controlling these diseases is to control the insect-carriers as is done in the case of malaria.

The Enteroviruses

The Enteroviruses are very small, being only one-thirtieth of the size of a staphylococcus. They inhabit the human alimentary canal and are transmitted from person to person.

Poliomyelitis virus is the cause of acute anterior poliomyelitis. There are three types, I, II and III, and there is no cross-protective immunity between them. The paralytic form of the disease is marked by muscular paralysis, encephalitis and aseptic meningitis. Many people infected with poliovirus suffer only a mild febrile illness.

Coxsackie viruses (about 25 types) cause meningitis, skin rashes, herpetic sore throat, febrile illnesses with pleurodynia, mild paralyses and occasionally myocarditis.

ECHO (*Enteric Cytopathogenic Human Orphan*) *viruses* (about 28 types) cause meningitis, skin rashes, respiratory infections, diarrhoea and mild paralysis.

Poliovirus infections may be severe and fatal, whereas

coxsackie and ECHO virus infections are usually mild and rarely fatal. Killed poliovirus is now used effectively to immunize against poliomyelitis. At present it is advisable to have three or possibly four courses at intervals of a few years, beginning in early childhood.

Herpes Simplex Virus

The herpes simplex virus, about one-twelfth the size of a staphylococcus, is the cause of the herpes around the mouth, often seen in patients with another infection, particularly pneumococcal pneumonia. Many people harbour the virus without experience of herpetic blisters. In the newborn or in older infants, herpes simplex virus may cause severe and fatal illness.

The Adenoviruses

The adenoviruses, which are as small as the poliovirus, inhabit human adenoids and tonsils and there are many types. They usually cause febrile respiratory illnesses, such as severe colds, but sometimes produce a 'gravelly' sore throat and conjunctivitis. The latter form of illness is called pharyngoconjunctival fever. One type of adenovirus caused an epidemic of conjunctivitis in Glasgow shipyards a few years ago.

Miscellaneous Viruses

The virus of *infective hepatitis* (*virus A*).

The virus of *homologous serum jaundice* (*virus B*).

Though the virus of infective hepatitis has never been isolated, the disease has been transmitted to human volunteers. Homologous serum jaundice is transmitted by transfused blood of donors who harbour the virus.

Other miscellaneous viruses include the viruses which cause rabies, measles and rubella.

Common Cold

Viruses causing these conditions have been isolated but not enough is yet known about them to fit them into any group.

Presumptive Virus Diseases

Presumptive virus diseases include infectious mononucleosis (glandular fever) and encephalitis lethargica (sleeping sickness).

Infectious mononucleosis may be the clinical result of an infection with one of several different viruses. Encephalitis lethargica has not occurred in epidemic form for over thirty years so there has been no opportunity to try out newest methods of virus isolation in this disease.

Some viruses such as the arboviruses (p. 109) always cause encephalitis; it may also be caused occasionally by many other viruses, namely influenza, mumps, measles, herpes simplex, vaccinia, coxsackie, ECHO and rabies viruses.

10 BACTERICIDES

JUST as organisms vary in the factors and conditions necessary for their growth, so they differ in their response to adverse conditions both physical and chemical. Some are killed easily by short exposure to a relatively low temperature, some, like the *Clostridium tetani,* still live after a long exposure to a high temperature. Some organisms are relatively susceptible to one type of killing agent, but resistant to another. The sensitivity of an organism to a killing agent is known as the organism's innate susceptibility and it depends upon many factors.

The bacterial kingdom with which the medical microbiologist is concerned can be divided into two parts, this division being based on the Gram stain, as described in Chapter 8. The ability to retain the dye which is shown by the Gram positive organisms obviously reflects a very different chemical constitution, and the Gram positive organisms are different in their response to killing agents from the Gram negative organisms. The Gram positive group includes a subgroup of organisms which are difficult to kill and which are at the same time highly dangerous to man in certain circumstances. They are the spore-bearing group to which *Cl. tetani, Bacillus anthracis* and *Cl. botulinum* belong.

When assessing a killing agent, the innate susceptibility of the organism it is desired to kill must be considered, and there are other factors which will influence the action of the killing agent:

1. The time necessary for action.

2. The concentration of killing agent.
3. The optimum acidity, or alkalinity for activity of killing agent.
4. The physical state of the material from which it is necessary to remove the bacteria; protein, blood, pus, mucus and dirt act as a protective coat for the bacteria and limit the action of many killing agents.
5. Antagonistic substances neutralizing the activity of the killing agent.
6. Impurities diluting the agent.
7. Inactivation of the agent by time.

The Choice of Killing Agents

Choosing a killing agent or bactericide for a particular purpose is a relatively simple matter if the contaminating organism is known. If a child has scarlet fever, the haemolytic streptococcus must be removed from his toys by some killing agent before the toys are played with by other children. The innate susceptibility of the haemolytic streptococcus is known and the choice of killing agent is wide, the limiting factor being the size and material to be disinfected. The particular process is designed to remove the streptococcus, which is a relatively susceptible organism; it will not remove other more resistant organisms which may be present on the toys, that is to say the toys are not necessarily made sterile or free from all organisms. In this case sterility is not essential; it would be impossible to keep toys sterile.

The choice of the killing agent to be used against the streptococcus in the patient, however, is governed by another limiting factor. The agent must be poisonous to the pathogenic organism in concentrations which are not harmful to the patient.

Materials or instruments which are to be introduced into the body, or which touch sites from which pathogenic organisms can get into the body, must be made completely sterile and free from all organisms. We have seen that the air and dust contain large numbers of organisms which being light and small can be wafted in air currents for long distances. It is not possible to know what organisms are present unless extensive bacteriological tests are done. To be on the safe side, therefore, all materials and instruments to be introduced into the body must be submitted to rigorous sterilizing techniques. The choice of killing agents in these cases is limited to those physical or chemical agents which will kill the most resistant organisms. Sterilization techniques should be checked at frequent intervals using one of the spore-bearing organisms as a test organism. If this can still grow after the sterilizing process the latter is inefficient and any equally resistant organisms which may have been present on the treated instruments or material will be living and a source of danger.

The Principles of Sterility

Bacteria were first seen under the microscope nearly 300 years ago, but it is only a little more than 100 years since contagion was linked with bacteriological contamination and cleanliness was first recognized as a preventive measure.

Soap and water was first used in 1847 by Semmelweiss deliberately to disinfect hands and instruments in surgical procedures. Since then ordinary social cleanliness has come to be recognized as of the first importance in the prevention of disease, because although soap and water do not make the instruments and hands bacteria-free, they do remove dirt and grease which act as binding agents for the bacteria. As the dirt and grease are washed off by soap, or by modern detergents, many bacteria are washed off as well.

Killing agents can be divided into two main groups, the physical agents and the chemical agents.

Physical Methods of Killing Bacteria

The physical methods of killing bacteria include:

Heat. Heat is the method of choice for the killing of bacteria on the majority of contaminated articles, and this may be applied as moist heat or dry heat.

Moist Heat. Moist heat in the form of steam under pressure circulating in an autoclave is the routine method of sterilization for all cotton fabrics such as gowns and theatre dressings, for rubber and for metals.

In many hospitals dressing drums or boxes, opened to allow steam to penetrate, have been replaced by specially made cardboard boxes which allow steam to penetrate but keep bacteria out. Now, as Central Sterile Supply Departments (CSSD) are being set up in an increasing number of hospitals or hospital groups, the trend is for dressings and appliances to be packed in specially prepared paper wrappings and inserted into imporous paper bags. Waterproof paper can replace rubber in the packs and paper towels replace cotton ones, whilst various types of synthetic dressings are being experimented with to replace gauze and wool. Ward sterilizers have disappeared where dressings are prepared centrally and only a clean dressing trolley has to be supplied by the ward. When this method is used, the paper containers are hung on the trolley and filled with the soiled dressings, which are then disposed of. Used instruments may be returned to a second bag and returned to the CSSD. The aim of this change is to produce better aseptic practice and it also reduces dramatically the time taken to prepare a dressing trolley.

The Autoclave. Most hospital autoclaves consist of a

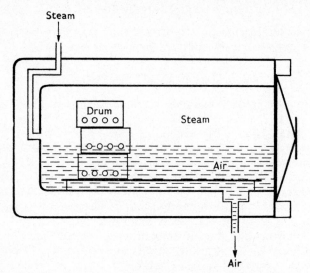

FIG. 36.—REMOVAL OF AIR FROM AN AUTOCLAVE BY DOWN-
WARD DISPLACEMENT.

THE DRUMS SHOWN MAY OF COURSE BE BOXES RATHER THAN
DRUMS.

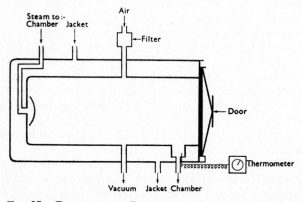

FIG. 37.—DIAGRAMMATIC REPRESENTATION OF AN AUTOCLAVE.

Figs. 36 and 37 are reproduced by kind permission of Longmans Green Ltd., from
Bacteriology and Immunity for Nurses by Ronald Hare.

horizontal cylinder with double walls and a hinged door at one end. Steam can be admitted both to the cylinder and to the jacket surrounding it. The articles to be sterilized are placed in the cylinder and after the door has been closed the air is either pumped out by means of a vacuum pump or is driven out by the incoming steam. All the air must be removed and replaced by steam if sterilization is to be complete.

After a stipulated time at a stipulated pressure, the steam inside the cylinder is pumped out in order to prevent its condensing and to avoid wetting the articles that have been sterilized. The heat from the steam-heated walls of the cylinder will thereafter assist the drying process.

Failure to get adequate sterilization by this means is rare, provided the apparatus is in the charge of a competent technician who understands the mechanism. Gauges, which may be checked by a chart, record temperature and pressure. The most frequent causes of failure are faulty autoclaves and inadequate penetration of steam. Sterilization should be checked at frequent intervals by packing pieces of lint or string impregnated with spore-bearing organisms in bottles or tubes in the centre of the containers. Failure of these organisms to grow after treatment and subsequent incubation means that the treatment was adequate and sterilization satisfactory. Brown's tubes are in use in most hospitals as a routine check. These contain waxes which change colour from red to green after being subjected to a known temperature for a known time. Another alternative is the Bowie-Dick autoclave tape test (pp. 72, 73).

Great advances have been made in the manufacture and design of autoclaves, and with the modern high vacuum, high temperature machine able to sterilize at 134° C (273° F), actual sterilizing time has been reduced to $3\frac{1}{2}$ minutes and the whole process need only take

16 minutes. The newest developments include fully automatic push button controls, each initiating a different sterilizing cycle suited to the materials to be sterilized, e.g. porous loads such as dressings, instruments

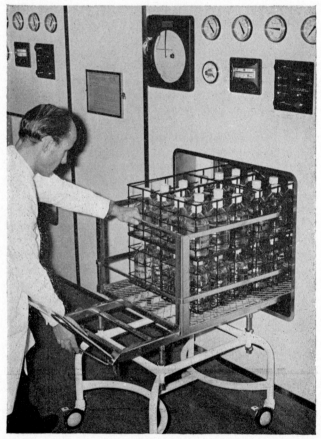

FIG. 38

and utensils needing quick drying, or the special sterilizing of bottled fluids (Fig. 38).

Another important advance is the automatic loading and unloading of equipment so that the unsterilized articles go directly from a packing and load preparation room into the autoclave, emerging from the sterilization process in a sterile goods store room. A suitable layout for one of these modern units, the Automotoclave (British Sterilizer Co), is shown in Fig. 39.

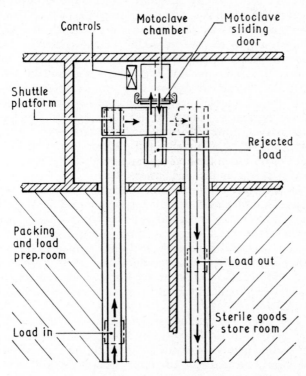

FIG. 39.—LAYOUT FOR A MODERN STERILIZING UNIT.

Against the initial expense of installation must be placed the reduction of possible sources of infection and the saving in manpower. One further point is that the modern machines incorporate devices for rejecting any load which is inadequately sterilized for whatever reason, i.e. pressure failure, air leak or any other factor (Fig. 39).

Sterilization by boiling water is still a convenient method for emergency home use. The time of 5 minutes boiling usually given is not, however, enough to ensure the killing of spores if these are present. It is a possible method of sterilizing all clean instruments, or trays, bowls and receivers, provided they are carefully cleansed and rinsed to remove all soiled material because the binding power of blood and pus serves to protect the organisms. This method has the disadvantage that sterilized instruments are wet and syringes treated in this way are unsuitable for vene-puncture or lumbar punctures; moreover, fluids for injection become diluted. Nowadays, however, even district nurses are often supplied with sterile packs and disposable syringes and needles for use in the home. Undoubtedly this is time and labour saving and is much safer.

Where ward sterilizers are still in use failure to kill organisms which do not form spores is usually due to human error, the apparatus is not completely immersed because the water has evaporated, or utensils are too closely packed, or the water had not returned to boiling point when timing was started. Other faults may be a badly fitting sterilizer lid or one that cannot close due to overloading so that steam escapes and reduces the efficacy of the boiling.

Dry Heat. Sixty minutes in a hot air oven at a temperature of 150° to 160° C kills spore-bearing organisms and this is the method of choice for sterilization of hardened glassware, particularly laboratory glassware, and some metals. The temperature in stainless steel ovens can be raised to 300° C. Rubber, many chemicals, plastics and cloth will not stand these high temperatures and cannot be sterilized in this way. Heat in an oven does not penetrate very well and failures may be due to uneven distribution of heat. Modern ovens sometimes have two doors, one opening from the working area and, on the opposite side, a second opening into the clean laboratory. (Fig. 40). Glass doors and thermometers visible from either side make for easy observation.

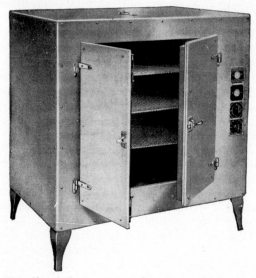

FIG. 40.—A DOUBLE-ENTRY STERILIZING OVEN.

Pasteurization. Pasteurization is the method of heat treatment of milk to make it safe for human consumption by removal of pathogenic bacteria such as typhoid bacilli, streptococci or tubercle bacilli which are frequently carried in milk; it is not a method of sterilization, but those organisms which remain after pasteurization are harmless when ingested.

There are two methods of pasteurization in common use in this country. The Holder process consisting of raising the temperature of the milk to 145° to 150° F (63° to 66° C) and keeping it there for 30 minutes, and then cooling quickly to 55° F (13° C) or below. The second method, the High Temperature Short Time method, keeps the milk at a temperature of not less than 161° F (72° C) for 20 seconds followed by cooling quickly to 55° F (13° C) or below. The Holder method can be adapted to use in the ward kitchen by standing a covered jug in continuously boiling water for 30 minutes and then plunging it into a basin of cold water.

Pasteurization removes the pathogenic bacteria in milk, with the advantage over boiling, which also sterilizes the milk, that it does not alter the taste unpleasantly.

Cold. Freezing as a method of killing bacteria is not satisfactory for ordinary use because the survival rate of organisms in low temperatures varies considerably. Refrigeration is, however, an excellent method for preserving food, sera etc., when the temperature is kept at about 4° C. Organisms are not killed by this method but they do not multiply. Perishable goods should be placed in the refrigerator immediately. If they are allowed to stay in a warm atmosphere for several hours organisms present in them will have a chance of multiplying and refrigeration after this time will be useless. Preformed toxins are not destroyed by refrigeration and no amount of cooling after they have been formed will make the food safe to eat (see Clostridia pp. 82, 172).

Drying. Many organisms are killed by drying, and this factor limits the natural spread of many diseases. Spores, however, can withstand remaining dry for many months or even years and, as a practical method of killing bacteria, drying is unsatisfactory.

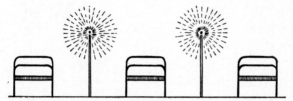

FIG. 41.—DIAGRAM OF A METHOD OF USING ULTRA-VIOLET LAMPS ON GLASS SCREENS TO PREVENT THE PASSAGE OF INFECTION BETWEEN BEDS.

Ultra-violet Light. Many of the vegetative forms of bacteria are killed by ultra-violet light but they vary in their susceptibility. Ultra-violet rays as a means of sterilization for instruments or materials are not practical but they have been tried for air disinfection in hospital wards in an attempt to keep down cross-infection. To get an effective concentration of rays, however, is very expensive and the rays are easily screened by glass and other materials. Some of the newer hospitals have barriers of ultra-violet light across the doorways between the main side wards to limit the spread of infection.

X-rays. Bacteria, like other rapidly multiplying cells, are killed by concentrations of X-rays, which in smaller doses alter the bacteria without killing them. X-rays, because of their effect on all living cells, are dangerous and as a means of sterilization or disinfection are unsuitable for routine use.

Gamma radiation or high energy ionizing irradiation is a form of radiant heat with high penetrating power and it is possible to obtain prepacked disposable catheters which have been sterilized by this form of heat at the Atomic Energy Research Establishment.

Physical Methods of Killing Bacteria

	Time	Strength	Penetration	Causes of Failure	Survival of Tetanus Spores	Suitability	Apparatus Required	Disadvantages
Heat — Moist	3½ min steam under 20 lb pressure and high vacuum	134° C / 275° F	Good	Failure of steam to penetrate. Faulty autoclave	Killed	All theatre dressings, also rubber, metal	Autoclave	Unsuitable for glass
	5 min boiling	100° C / 212° F	Good	Evaporation	Not certain	All clean ward instruments	Covered pan. Water must cover articles	Unsuitable for soiled material
Heat — Dry	60 min	150°–160° C / 302°–320° F	Poor	Uneven heat	Killed	Glass. Some metals	Oven	Unsuitable for rubber and many chemicals
Cold	Slow	−10° C to −120° C	Poor	Freezing points too variable	Variable	For preserving food, sera etc.	Refrigerator	—
Drying	Slow	—	Poor	Time uncertain	Spores survive	Impracticable for ordinary work	Hot air oven	Expensive
Ultra-violet light	Variable	Variable	Variable	Easily screened	Variable	do.	Lamp	do.
X-rays	Variable	Variable	Good	Easily screened	Variable	do.	X-ray apparatus	Dangerous
Gamma rays	—	—	Good	—	Killed	do.	Atomic energy	—

Moist heat is the method of choice, either autoclaving or boiling, as moist heat readily coagulates the protein of an organism.

Chemical Methods of Killing Bacteria

The word disinfectant is a term reserved for the gross cell poisons like phenol (carbolic) which destroy both bacterial and tissue cells by virtue of their power to denature or destroy protein. Their destructive action is non-specific, so that disinfectants can only be used to sterilize apparatus and are too dangerous to living cells to be used on skin or internally. Weaker poisons which destroy bacteria but do not cause much damage to body cells are often called antiseptics, and substances belonging to this group, like acriflavine, can be used on the skin with safety, although they are too toxic to be used internally.

Such definitions of disinfectants and antiseptics are, however, not strict definitions because in many cases the cell-destroying power of a substance depends upon its strength and the length of time for which it is used. Generally speaking, disinfectants are used to sterilize inanimate objects, and antiseptics, which are less efficient and less toxic, are used to clean skin and to preserve sterility once this has been achieved by other methods.

Up till 1881 there were no known substances which could be used to destroy an invading organism within the body because the known disinfectants and antiseptics were non-selective in their action and destroyed bacteria and host cells to the same degree. In 1881 Koch tried experimentally to abort anthrax in guinea pigs, using mercuric chloride. He aborted the anthrax but the antiseptic killed the animals.

In 1904 Ehrlich cured experimental trypanosomiasis (sleeping sickness) by using a dye, trypan red, and in 1910 the arsenical compound salversan was found to cure some protozoal and spirochaetal diseases while preserving the patient. It was used successfully to treat syphilis for many years. This was virtually the extent of specific drug therapy (chemotherapy) for infectious diseases until 1935.

Chemotherapeutic Agents

In 1935 Domagk reported some success against bacterial diseases due to the haemolytic streptococcus with a drug of the sulphonamide group. This was the beginning of modern chemotherapy. It was subsequently found that in the body this drug was converted into para-aminobenzene sulphonamide (or sulphanilamide) and this was the active part of the substance.

Since 1935 various other drugs have been synthesized to give a wider range of activity against more bacteria, greater potency, less toxicity, and different physico-chemical properties, but the action of the whole group is fundamentally the same, depending on the sulphanila-mide content. The action of these drugs is bacteriostatic, rather than bactericidal. The organisms are prevented from growing and multiplying and the normal defence mechanisms of the body are enabled to deal with the infection. In 1940 Wood suggested that the sulphona-mides produce their effect by interfering with some important metabolic pathway of the organism.

We have seen that bacteria vary enormously in the nutritive material which they can use for building up into bacterial protoplasm and enzymes and for breaking down to provide the energy necessary for this synthesis. Some organisms provided with atmospheric nitrogen and carbon can synthesize complex bacterial proteins by an enormous number of chemical changes, each change being catalyzed or brought about by a specific enzyme, the process forming a chain of reactions culminating in new bacterial bodies. Loss of an enzyme along this chain of reactions will cause a break in the chain and growth will stop unless the substance is provided in the form of another material, chemically 'nearer' in the chain of the reactions to the bacterial protoplasm, in which case the need for the missing enzyme is eliminated. A substance or chemical group which is necessary for growth of a particular organism is known as an essential metabolite for that organism.

All bacteria which are sensitive to the sulphonamides, and that is a wide range of organisms, require as an essential metabolite para-aminobenzoic acid. This substance is very similar to sulphanilamide, but sulphanilamide is not biologically active and it cannot take the place of the essential metabolite in the chain of reactions. It is, however, sufficiently similar to react with the enzyme of the bacterial body which uses para-aminobenzoic acid. Once the enzyme has reacted with the drug the chain of reactions becomes blocked and growth cannot take place.

In order to produce an effective concentration in the blood, a high dose is given initially, and the dose is subsequently reduced to a maintenance level which ensures a high ratio of sulphonamide to para-amino benzoic acid.

If the organism is to survive in a medium flooded with sulphanilamide it must either make its own para-aminobenzoic acid from simpler substances or adopt a chain of reactions by-passing the reaction needing para-aminobenzoic acid. Both these courses are possible if the bacteria are given sufficient time; they can be trained to do without the essential metabolite and once this resistant strain has been produced, further sulphonamide treatment is useless. It is essential therefore to prevent pathogenic organisms from making these metabolic adjustments, and this is done by flooding the tissues with a sulphonamide. Inadequate therapy and small doses are dangerous, because once a resistant strain has been produced, there is evidence to suggest that even in a different host this strain remains resistant.

Para-aminosalicylic acid (PAS) stands in the same relationship to salicylic acid as the sulphonamides do to para-aminobenzoic acid. The growth of virulent tubercle bacilli is stimulated by salicylic acid and inhibited by the closely related substance para-amino-salicylic acid.

The Woods-Fildes hypothesis of bacteriostasis by blocking systems has far reaching implications; as more becomes known about the normal metabolic pathways of pathogenic organisms it should be possible to select drugs which are known to interfere with the various reactions, and this method of searching for chemo-therapeutic substances is a rational one.

Antibiotics

Naturally occurring antibacterial substances are known as antibiotics. It has been known for many years that substances produced by various groups of bacteria or moulds will inhibit the growth of other groups of organisms. Many of these substances are also toxic to animal tissues but a few are sufficiently selective in their action against microorganisms to be used as therapeutic agents. It was not, however, until 1929 that the full importance of these substances was recognized.

Penicillin. In 1928, Fleming noticed that colonies of staphylococci were 'dissolved' round a mould of *Penicillin notatum* which was growing by accident on a culture plate. From this mould Florey later extracted the active substance penicillin, the pure form of which is now known as benzylpenicillin or penicillin G. It is supplied as the sodium or potassium salt and is also known as soluble or crystalline penicillin.

Penicillin is very selective in its action and in general it may be said that the Gram positive cocci and bacilli, the pathogenic Gram negative cocci and the spirochaetes are sensitive, while the Gram negative rods and the viruses are penicillin-resistant.

Those organisms which are resistant to penicillin are resistant either because they can grow unharmed in penicillin or because they themselves produce a substance which destroys penicillin. It is for this reason that treatment by penicillin of a mixed infection due to a sensitive and a resistant organism so often fails. One sees it frequently in varicose ulcers, or external ear infections. The primary causative organism is sensitive, but the lesion becomes secondarily infected with a penicillin-destroying organism.

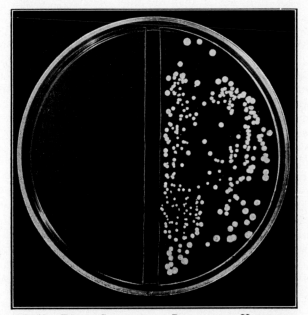

FIG. 42.—TEST OF SENSITIVITY TO PENICILLIN BY HALF-PLATE METHOD. THE AGAR ON THE LEFT WAS INOCULATED BUT THE PENICILLIN IN IT HAS DESTROYED THE ORGANISMS.

In all sensitive cultures there are a few organisms which are relatively more resistant than the rest; these arise naturally. In the presence of concentrations of penicillin sufficient to kill the majority, this minority are not killed and they multiply; in this way a resistant strain is established. Since the regular use of penicillin the number of resistant strains of some organisms, particularly staphylococci, has enormously increased; this is why chemotherapy should be reserved for serious infections.

Penicillin is non-toxic, so that dosage cannot be too high. It is, however, easily inactivated, the newer, purer preparations less so than the older ones. Such things as heat, acids, alkalis, alcohol, metals, oxidizing agents, disinfectants and time readily destroy its potency. The dry salt of benzylpenicillin is, however, stable at room temperature. Because of its inactivation by acids, benzylpenicillin is partially destroyed in the stomach, but it may successfully be given by mouth if in sufficiently large doses. For severe infections, however, it must be given by intramuscular injection. It is now considered bad therapy to prescribe small doses of penicillin for local application, e.g. in toothpaste, chewing gum or lozenges which may encourage the development of resistant strains of bacteria and make the patient allergic to the drug.

Penicillin diffuses rapidly through the tissues and an adequate blood level is reached within 15 minutes of an intramuscular injection; the excretion rate through the kidneys is also rapid so that however large a dose of crystalline penicillin is given the level falls quickly, and after 3 hours another dose must be given if an adequate level is to be maintained.

Three-hourly injections were wearisome to the patient in hospital and extremely difficult in domiciliary cases. Various new preparations of the drug have, however, been introduced under proprietary names, the drug being suspended in a substance from which it is released slowly into the surrounding tissues. Large quantities are given intramuscularly and penicillin is gradually released, so that an adequate blood level, i.e. amount of the drug in the blood stream, can be maintained for 24 hours after a single injection

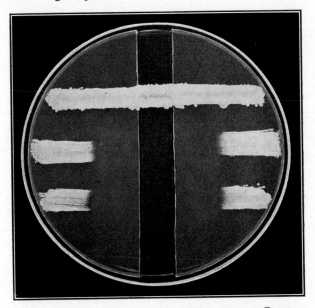

FIG. 43.—TEST OF SENSITIVITY TO PENICILLIN BY GUTTER-PLATE METHOD. NOTE THE AREA CLEARED OF ORGANISM NEAREST TO THE PENICILLIN-CONTAINING AGAR STRIP.

More recently, the basic nucleus of penicillin has been isolated and it is now possible to produce semi-synthetic modifications. These include phenoxymethyl-penicillin or penicillin V, Broxil (phenethicillin), Celbenin (methicillin) and Penbritin (ampicillin). Broxil is an antibiotic which is grown initially as a mould and modified chemically; therefore it is semi-synthetic. It is used orally, 125 or 250 mg tablets 6-hourly will maintain high blood levels. Celbenin, a similarly produced antibiotic, can be used against penicillin-resistant strains of staphylococci because it is not inactivated by penicillinase. It must be freshly prepared and kept in the refrigerator. It is given in doses of 1 g intramuscularly 4-hourly for 3 days, then 6-hourly for 3 days. Penbritin is another new penicillin which is effective against Gram negative organisms such as Salmonella, Shigella and *Escherichia coli* in doses of 750 mg 8-hourly.

Streptomycin. Since the discovery of penicillin there have been numerous other antibacterial substances produced from soil bacteria, notably the streptomyces group of which streptomycin was one of the first.

Streptomycin inhibits the growth of nearly all pathogenic organisms with the exception of the spore-bearing organisms, fungi, viruses and rickettsiae; it has therefore the advantage over penicillin of inhibiting the Gram negative rods including the coli-typhoid-dysentery group, and also the *Mycobacterium tuberculosis*.

Streptomycin is given by intramuscular injection because, although it is more stable than penicillin, it is not absorbed through the gut. Its excretion by the kidneys is not so rapid as penicillin and adequate blood levels can be maintained for 6 to 12 hours after a single injection.

Streptomycin produces serious vestibular disturbances, and sometimes deafness after prolonged treatment and less serious toxic symptoms such as nausea and vomiting make it an unpopular drug with patients.

Streptomycin is the most active agent in use against tubercle bacilli, and the best results have been obtained in tuberculous meningitis and in acute, generalized or miliary tuberculosis. The main difficulty of streptomycin therapy in tuberculosis and in other diseases is the emergence of streptomycin-resistant strains. For this reason it is now always given in combination with either para-aminosalicylate (PAS) or isoniazid, which prevent the emergence of resistant strains.

Streptomycin has also proved useful in urinary tract infections, particularly those caused by the Gram negative bacilli.

Chloramphenicol (Chloromycetin), also produced by some strains of streptomyces, is now produced synthetically. It is active against the Gram positive cocci, Gram negative bacilli, the organism of relapsing fever, the rickettsiae and some of the larger viruses. The rickettsiae, a group of organisms producing typhus, respond to treatment with chloramphenicol. Other virus diseases which respond are psittacosis and atypical virus pneumonia. Diseases due to the minute viruses are not improved.

Chloramphenicol has the advantage of being absorbed from the gut and there are reports of good results in the treatment of enteric fever. The main limitation to its use is its liability to cause blood dyscrasias, in particular a fatal aplastic anaemia.

The Tetracyclines. The main broad spectrum antibiotics in current use are the tetracyclines (aureomycin, tetramycin and achromycin).

Chlortetracycline (Aureomycin). This antibiotic is produced by another strain of *Streptomyces*. It is well absorbed by mouth and the oral preparations available are stable when kept at moderate room temperature. Injection solutions are less stable and should be freshly prepared. It is active against the Gram negative bacilli and the Gram positive and Gram negative cocci. Certain Gram negative bacilli, such as the *Proteus* and *Pseudomonas* groups are, however, relatively resistant.

Chlortetracycline causes severe nausea and some diarrhoea in many patients; this can be reduced by giving the drug in milk. **Oxytetracycline** (Terramycin) has a similar range and toxicity to Aureomycin.

Both chloramphenicol and the tetracyclines are drugs with a wide range of bacteriostatic power, so that their administration inhibits the growth of both pathogens and non-pathogenic organisms which are normally present on the healthy mucous membranes. These non-pathogens play a complex important part in the metabolism of the body. Just how important this part is, is not yet fully realized. The bacterial flora of the gut and respiratory tract is profoundly altered after giving chloromycetin and chlortetracycline, and this change produces deleterious effects. There may be vitamin B deficiency associated with the destruction of intestinal bacteria, which produces symptoms of vulval and anal irritation, and there may be vesiculopapular eruptions on the mucous membranes.

Among the other antibiotics which are now generally available, **neomycin** is active against a wide range of bacteria although it produces toxic signs in the kidneys and ears. **Terramycin** has a similar range and toxicity to Aureomycin. **Tetracycline** (Achromycin) is active against Gram positive and Gram negative organisms and *Rickettsia orientalis* (scrub typhus). It is well absorbed in oral administration and has now largely replaced Aureomycin and Terramycin in routine clinical use.

More antibiotic substances are being discovered rapidly, and it is becoming apparent that these substances, which are so powerful, have disadvantages as well as advantages. Too little is yet known of the relationship between the metabolism of the normal bacterial flora and the host metabolism, and the administration of one antibiotic may produce an incidental effect on the other organisms on the mucous membranes, with the development of an antibiotic-fast strain of bacteria which may last for many bacterial generations.

To sum up, it is true to say that there are antibiotics now available to deal with the whole pathogenic bacterial kingdom, and the future course of bacterial disease may well depend upon the proper use of the right ones.

Antibiotic treatment cannot replace antiserum treatment in the toxaemias such as tetanus, gas gangrene and diphtheria; the two lines of treatment must go together. The antibiotic inhibits the growth of the organism, but does not neutralize the preformed toxin. The treatment of the virus diseases, however, other than the diseases caused by the large ones, is another matter. Their position, intracellular and out of reach of the tissue fluids, and the fact that their metabolism is so intimately bound up with that of the host metabolism, has so far made many of them immune to available chemotherapeutic agents and antibiotics.

Disinfectants and Antiseptics

The chemical agents used as disinfectants and antiseptics are employed against bacteria infecting inanimate objects and on the human skin, and in wounds and body cavities, such as the mouth, throat and vagina, which cannot be treated by heat. In these cases chemicals which would be injurious if taken by mouth can be used, but in each case the substance must be carefully chosen to suit the purpose for which it is needed. Disinfectants are chemicals which kill bacteria and are today often referred to as bactericides. Antiseptics are less strong: they do not kill bacteria, but prevent their growth and multiplication; nowadays they are sometimes referred to as bacteriostatics because they bring bacterial growth to a standstill without actually killing the organism.

Disinfectants and antiseptics in common use today include:

(1) The halogens, e.g. iodine, chlorine and providone-iodine
(2) Heavy metals, e.g. mercury, silver
(3) The phenols and cresols, coal tar derivatives
(4) Chloroxylenols, e.g. Roxenol, Dettol
(5) Cationic detergents, such as cetrimide (CTAB or Cetavlon), Roccal and Savlon
(6) Oxydizing agents, e.g. peroxide of hydrogen and permanganate of potash
(7) Acridines, e.g. acriflavine
(8) Aniline dyes, e.g. gentian violet, brilliant green

The Halogens. These are non-metallic elements, so-called because they produce salts, salts which are present in sea water. They include iodine, chlorine and bromine, and of these iodine and chlorine are useful sources of disinfectants and antiseptics. *Iodine* is derived from seaweed; it is insoluble in water, but will dissolve in a solution of potassium iodide. It may be made up as 'tincture of iodine', at $2\frac{1}{2}\%$ solution, in 70% alcohol with potassium iodide; this may be painted on the skin to disinfect superficial bruises and grazes, though it causes severe smarting pain; or diluted 7 g to a litre for arm baths or vaginal douching. Iodine may be used to purify the skin for operation, but for this purpose iodine $2\frac{1}{2}\%$, in rectified spirit should be used, as the tincture gives off an irritating vapour which will affect the surgeon's eyes as he bends over the site of operation. Betadine (providone-iodine) is a newer form of iodine preparation for disinfecting the skin; it has the advantages over other forms of being less irritating, the stain is more easily removable by washing and the bactericidal effect lasts longer.

Chlorine is an irritating, poisonous gas, greenish in colour, which was used in chemical warfare in the 1914-18 war because of the fatal results which followed the breathing of this gas. Chlorine compounds are, however, useful in medicine. Chlorinated lime or bleaching powder is a valuable disinfectant for drains and excreta, and solutions are useful for disinfecting linen. Solutions derived from this include eusol, Dakin's solution, electrolytic sodium hypochlorite solution (or Milton) and chloramine-T or Chloros. Eusol and Dakin's were solutions discovered during the 1914-18 war in the search for antiseptics which could disinfect a wound without injuring the tissues, before the discovery of the sulphonamides and antibiotics. Eusol was first produced by the research department of Edinburgh University—hence the name E(dinburgh) U(niversity) Sol(lution). It contains equal parts of chlorinated lime and boracic acid; it is alkaline in reaction and therefore somewhat irritating, but much less so than the mercurial salts which had previously been used for swabbing wounds. It is cheap to produce, but it is inactivated by light and must be kept in dark bottles. It should be used within three weeks after dispensing. Dakin's solution is similar, but also contains sodium bicarbonate, which enables it to dissolve sloughs. It is more stable, and it is similar in its properties and uses. Both of these solutions give off chlorine, which combines with proteins in the tissue cells and bacteria. Both are mildly antiseptic and non-toxic, and only slightly irritating. They can be used for irrigating wounds, and gauze soaked in these solutions can be placed in and over wounds. Surrounding skin should be covered with dry gauze, or may be protected by petroleum jelly, since the lotion may injure the skin because of its alkalinity.

Electrolytic sodium hypochlorite or Milton is another solution which sets free chlorine and may be used for washing wounds, for irrigation, and on dressings. It was used widely during the Second World War in the Bunyan-Stannard coated silk treatment of burns and wounds. It is non-toxic and produces little irritation at a strength of $2\frac{1}{2}$ to 5% solution.

Chloramine-T and Chloros are complicated organic compounds, with a strength of 12% active chlorine. They are useful as mouth washes, particularly in cases of operation or radium treatment of the tongue, protecting the tissues from septic infection more satisfactorily than other mild antiseptics, suitable for contact with mucous membrane and skin. Chloros 5%, for 1 hour can be used to disinfect the faeces of a patient with poliomyelitis.

Salts of Heavy Metals. Mercurial salts, particularly perchloride, biniodide and oxycyanides of mercury were freely used in the past as disinfectants and antiseptics. They are absorbed on to the surface of bacteria and then penetrate and kill them. Their bactericidal power is lessened by the presence of serum, pus and blood and other organic matter. They coagulate protein and so do not penetrate it quickly. They are highly toxic. In low concentrations water-soluble salts such as *perchloride of mercury*, at a strength of 1 in 1000 to 1 in 8000, are effective disinfectants for many purposes, but they irritate skin, tarnish metals and become relatively useless when mixed with organic matter such as faeces, sputum and pus. They are chiefly used today as compounds containing a small quantity of mercury only, for example *phenylmercuric acetate* or *nitrate*; these are used for the chemical sterilization of delicate instruments such as cystoscopes, which cannot be exposed to heat, strength 1 in 10,000; for skin preparation, strength 1 in

2000 to 1 in 5000; and for douching, 1 in 3000. They should not be used for disinfectant baths, as they coagulate discharge and prevent its escape. Yellow mercuric oxide 1% is the antiseptic in Golden Eye Ointment.

The Phenols and Cresol. These are derivatives of coal tar. Phenol or carbolic acid is interesting historically as it was the disinfectant used by Lord Lister to prevent contamination of wounds. Following Pasteur's discovery that all fermentation of sugar and starch was due to the growth of bacteria in them. Lister applied the principle, after experimentation, to surgery. In the days when surgeons wore old clothes, possibly splashed with blood and pus, when operating, and hands, instruments and bowls were merely washed between cases, he soaked his hands, instruments, dressing towels and bowls in carbolic solution 1 in 20. Under such conditions he opened the knee joint to remove a loose semilunar cartilage, and opened the abdomen. He incised tuber-culous abscesses, passing his scalpel through a square of muslin soaked in 1 in 20 carbolic lotion, which he called a 'guard'. For a time the air of the operating theatre was sprayed with a mist of carbolic lotion to prevent bacterial infection of the wound from the air, though he and his assistants suffered from carboluria as a result of it. When it was later discovered that heat could kill germs as effectively as carbolic and other disinfectants, the use of carbolic became gradually more and more restricted, but it had enabled Lister to prove that bacteria were the cause of sepsis and to carry out operations which his colleagues at the time believed would have fatal results. When in 1877 he came to King's College Hospital from Edinburgh and removed a slipped cartilage from the knee, contemporary surgeons in London expected the patient to die and were prepared to remove his name from the Medical Register of the General Medical Council on a charge of malpractice. To their surprise the operation wound healed by first intention and an important step had been taken in establishing the theory that sepsis was due to bacterial infection.

Phenol or *carbolic* in pure form is crystalline, but in strong solution (90%) produces a liquid, formerly known as 'pure carbolic' which is highly caustic, and is used to cauterize the appendix stump and corneal ulcers in surgery today. In 5% solution (1 in 20) it can be used to disinfect stools and sputum. Because of the conservatism in medical and nursing practice, it is still used in some institutions, since it is safe, although newer antiseptics either more efficient or less expensive should be substituted for it. It is useful in weak solution (1 in 80 to 1 in 100) as a mouth wash or gargle because it has also an anaesthetic effect. For this reason it may also be used in skin ointment to allay itching. Lysol, Jeyes' Fluid and Cyllin are saponified or emulsified solutions of coal tar derivatives (cresol and phenol). The soapy solutions will be curdled if added to hard water, in the same way that toilet and washing soaps are, but they will mix with distilled water. They are divided into the white preparations such as Jeyes, Izal and Lysol, and the black disinfectant fluids such as Cyllin. They are specially useful where large quantities of solution are required, for example to disinfect linen, bed pans and excreta. Black fluids must be suitably diluted before linen is put into them or they will stain it (strength 1 in 160). Cyllin properly prepared is good for soaking linen, as it does not coagulate protein and therefore does not set stains from discharges and excreta. This is because it does not contain phenol. Jeyes' Fluid and Izal are proprietary preparations which can be used for similar purposes; at a strength of 1 in 100 to 1 in 160 they are disinfectant if allowed to act for a sufficient length of time; at a strength of 1 in 320 they are antiseptic. Lysol contains cresol in a 25% soap solution. It is more expensive than cruder preparations such as Cyllin and should therefore be used with care. In strong solutions it is caustic and should be washed from skin or eyes immediately, if they are accidentally splashed. In solutions of 1 in 100 or 1 in 160 (7 ml to 1 litre of water) it is an effective disinfectant, dissolves albuminous discharges, reaching quickly the bacteria they contain, and is a useful cleansing agent for surgical baths. These may be swabbed with a gloved hand, using a swab on a stick or old pair of forceps, left for a few minutes and thoroughly rinsed. Lysol-Sudol has very largely replaced Lysol. Printol also belongs to the phenol group of bactericides. It is effective, 1 in 100, against a wide range of bacteria, e.g. pyogenic, coliform, salmonella and pseudomonas groups and is not inactivated by organic material. Its activity is increased by soaps and detergents and it is non-corrosive. It is not irritant to skin and at recommended dilutions does not destroy linen.

Hycolin, a synergetic mixture of synthetic phenols, is used in a 1% solution. It appears to destroy all pathogenic organisms except spores. It is effective in the presence of hard water, yeasts and blood serum. No bacterial resistance and no skin sensitivity (except possibly in phenol sensitives) has been shown to develop. Combined with hexachlorophene in a soap or cream it provides an excellent antiseptic for ward use. (Hands should be washed for two minutes.)

Chlorine Derivatives. Chlorocresol and chloroxylenol or Roxenol, derived from the action of chlorine on cresol and xylenol respectively, are useful disinfectants against streptococci (Dettol and Streph are proprietary preparations in this group). They are much less caustic than phenol or Lysol in strong solution. They are expensive and relatively ineffective, but are non-irritant and non-toxic in strong solutions. Dettol may be used as a liquid, cream or ointment for application to the skin, but it is ineffective against staphylococci. Dettol lotion may be used for douching in strength 1 in 160. Roxenol is one of the most widely used antiseptics in this group.

Cationic Detergents. Examples of these are cetrimide (cetyltrimethyl ammonium bromide), CTAB, or Cetavlon, a proprietary preparation, and Roccal (benzalkonium chloride 1%): these are cleansing agents. They dissolve sebum and grease and have a bactericidal action, but are not effective against *Bacillus pyocyaneus*. They are not compatible with soap so that the two must not be used together.

Some hospitals now use cetrimide 15% w/v plus chlorhexidine (Hibitane) 1·5% w/v in a mixture called Savlon for cleansing the skin. Hibitane 1% is also used after scrubbing up or hand washing either as a solution or a hand cream, particularly for obstetric purposes.

Phisohex, which contains chlorhexidine and Roccal is used in some hospitals as a skin disinfectant.

Oxidizing agents. These have a mild antiseptic action because of the oxygen they set free when in contact with organic matter. They include *hydrogen peroxide* and *potassium permanganate*. Hydrogen peroxide readily gives off oxygen and is dispensed as a solution, the strength of which is measured by the volume of oxygen given off compared with the volume of the lotion used. It is generally dispensed as a 10 to 20% solution (H_2O_2 10 vols. strength) i.e. the lotion gives off a volume of oxygen $\frac{1}{10}$ to $\frac{1}{5}$ the volume of the fluid. This effervescing property helps mechanically to bring pus up from a deep wound, to loosen any sloughs and help to bring them away. It should be used in small quantities, which should be allowed to effervesce in the wound or part so that none of its action is wasted. After giving off oxygen it becomes plain water, with no disinfectant property, so that it should not be left to lie in wounds or cavities. It may be followed by eusol or electrolytic sodium hypochlorite, if an antiseptic effect is to be left in the wound, or washed out with sterile normal saline solution and gently dried.

Potassium permanganate is a crystalline substance which produces a purplish fluid. If this has turned brown the oxygen has already been given off and the lotion is stale and has no disinfectant property. It has been used in weak solution for antiseptic baths, and vaginal douches, strength 1 in 5000, or as a gargle, 1 in 10,000. It is less used today, as newer remedies have largely replaced it.

The Acridines. These are a group of dyes also used in surgery to cleanse wounds and on dressings for open wounds. *Proflavine hemisulphate*, *Euflavine* and *aminacrine hydrochloride* are the preparations most often used today, as acriflavine is more irritating and less easily prepared. They are used strength 1 in 1000 in aqueous solution for swabbing wounds and on dressings and in alcoholic solution for preparation of the skin for operation. In aqueous solutions strength 1 in 10,000 they may be used for bladder washouts. They are non-irritant but more expensive than the drugs used for other disinfectant purposes and stain the skin temporarily.

The Aniline Dyes. These are derived from coal tar, and the ones mainly used are *gentian violet* and *brilliant green*; these may be used separately or combined in *Bonney's blue*, or in combination with proflavine as

Table of Some of the Chemical Agents Used as Disinfectants or Antiseptics

Chemical Group		Preparation Used	Strength	Use
Halogens	Iodine	Tincture of iodine	2½% in 70% alcohol	As a skin disinfectant
		Betadine antiseptic		As a skin disinfectant
	Chlorine	Chloros, Chloramine T.	12% active chlorine	For sterilizing of water supplies
		Sodium hypochlorite	12% active chlorine	For irrigation of cavities
		Milton	1:80 active chlorine	To disinfect baby bottles
		Dakin's Solution (stable)	15% active chlorine	
		Chloros	10%	For disinfecting excreta containing poliomyelitis virus
Metals	Mercury	Phenylmercuric nitrate	1:2000 aqueous and alcoholic	Bacteriostatic not bactericidal. Poor penetrating power and relatively ineffective.
		Merthiolate (Tincture)	1:1000	Used as skin antiseptic and fungicidal ointment
			1:10,000	eye lotion
Phenols		Phenol	1:20	For storing instruments
			1:80	Disinfecting linen for 12 hours
	Creso	Lysol	1:160	For disinfecting linen for 12 hours to 24 hours
			1:20	For cleaning infected baths
		Jeyes' Fluid	1:160	Relatively cheap disinfectants used for disinfecting linen for 12–24 hours. Used for cleaning floors in sanitary annexes. Never used on skin since they are corrosive
		Sanitas	1:80	
		White Cyllin		

Category	Preparation	Strength	Uses
Chloroxylenols	Roxenol Dettol Osyl Streph	Dispensed as 1:20 solution: used in strengths 1:140 1:160	Expensive and relatively ineffective For skin disinfection For douching
Cationic Detergents			
Cetyltrimethyl ammonium bromide	Cetrimide, CTAB, Cetavlon Roccal Savlon	1% 1:40 to 1:10 1:80 to 1:10 1:200 to 1:30	Useful for all purposes. Can be used on skin or instruments and utensils. Detergent action makes these substances good for removing grease and organic material
Oxydizing Agents	Hydrogen peroxide	10-20 vols.	For irrigation of cavities, for removal of pus or blood
Acridines			
Acriflavine	Proflavine hemisulphate	1:1000 { aqueous neutral alcoholic	Non-irritant skin disinfectants for wound swabbing and dressing
	Euflavine	1:1000 { aqueous acid alcoholic	
Aniline Dyes	Gentian violet	1%	For skin preparation before operation. Active against cocci, and used as a fungicide in skin treatments and in vaginal pessaries
	Triple dye	Gentian violet 0.2% Brilliant green 0.2% Proflavine hemisulphate 0.1%	For skin preparation before operation

'*triple dye*' for the treatment of burns. They are used strength 1 to 2% for skin purification after careful cleansing with a detergent.

Boracic acid is a mild antiseptic, non-irritating to delicate tissues such as the conjunctiva, and the mucous membranes lining the nose, mouth and bladder. It was widely used for irrigation and the rinsing of instruments coming into contact with these tissues, but its effect is so slight that it has been largely replaced by sterilized normal saline solution. Normal saline must be carefully protected from contamination before and during its use in surgical procedures.

Sterilization of Ward and Theatre Apparatus

Article	*Method of Choice*
Dressings Cotton Wool Bandages, Cloths and Towels used in Theatre	Autoclave at 15 lb pressure for 20 minutes or at 20 lb pressure for 10 minutes with pure steam or 3½ minutes in high vacuum autoclave.
Rubber Gloves (unless diposable)	Soak in cold water, wash in warm soapy water. Dry, examine, and powder. Autoclave at 6 lb pressure for 15 minutes. It is undesirable to use patched gloves in the theatre.
Rubber Catheters (unless disposable)	Wash thoroughly with cold followed by warm water, using Higginson's syringe. Boil in a covered boiler for 5 minutes, dry by rinsing through with ether, and put in airtight metal container with formalin tablets. 24 hours is sufficient to establish sterility; if the formalin container has a heated base 12 hours is sufficient. Catheters must be rinsed in sterile distilled water to remove formalin before use. Glutaraldehyde 2·5% in distilled water is a less toxic but more active alternative. It is not a stable solution and should be renewed fortnightly. *For all rubber goods see alternative p.166.*

Sterilization of Ward and Theatre Apparatus—*(cont.)*

Article	*Method of Choice*
Gum Elastic Catheters Ureteric Catheters	Clean in the same way as rubber catheters. Store in formalin.
Rubber and Mackintosh Sheets	Wash or scrub with detergent bactericide such as Savlon 1 in 200, Lysol 1 in 40 or Printol 1 in 100. Rinse, dry and powder and autoclave at 15 lb pressure for 20 minutes.
Metal Instruments	Scrub in soapy warm water or with a detergent. Autoclave at 15 lb pressure for 20 minutes or $3\frac{1}{2}$ minutes in high vacuum, high temperature autoclave, boil for 5 minutes in a covered boiler or use a hot air oven at a temperature of 160° C for 1 hour.
Glass and Metal Syringes	Autoclave at 15 lb for 15 minutes or reduced time in high vacuum, high temperature autoclave, or in a hot air oven at 160° C for 1 hour.
Needles	Autoclave at 15 lb pressure for 15 minutes or reduced time in high vacuum, high temperature autoclave.
Bowls and Basins	Boil 5 minutes in covered boiler or autoclave.
Crockery	Wash with detergent, e.g. Savlon 1 in 40 or Printol 1 in 100 and rinse well, or boil in a covered boiler for 5 minutes.
Wash Basins and Baths	Wash with detergent, bactericide, e.g. Savlon 0·5% (1 in 200), Lysol 1 in 40, cetrimide 1%, or Printol 1 in 100, followed by thorough rinsing.
Nailbrushes	Boil for 5 minutes at least daily, and use dry from a covered box.
Cystoscopes	If boilable, should be boiled for 5 minutes. Boiling will damage other types; these may be soaked in phenylmercuric nitrate 1 in 2000 for 20 minutes then rinsed well in sterile distilled water.

Sterilization of Ward and Theatre Apparatus—*(cont.)*

Article	*Method of Choice*
Plastic Apparatus	Polythene tubing, catheters, etc., may be boiled for 5 minutes. Clear plastic instruments used for diagnostic examination or for lighting internal cavities, e.g. Coldlite specula, retractors, auriscopes, may be boiled for 5 minutes, and wrapped up to prevent scratching. They must not be soaked in phenol, lysol or other acid disinfectants, as these make them cloudy and ineffective. Methylated or surgical spirit will also discolour them. They must not be put into an autoclave. They can be washed with cetrimide 1% solution, but must not lie in it.

Ward Kitchens

There is no place more important, whether in hospital or in the home, than the kitchen where the principles underlying the prevention of infection are concerned. Every source of infection can lead to the hands, and in addition coughing and sneezing in the kitchen can cause direct infection of food (Figs. 6-8 and Chapter 11).

Trained and student nurses should set themselves a high standard as regards the handling of such things as cups, glasses, silver cutlery and plates, and should never allow themselves to be guilty of such potentially dangerous habits as, for example, holding glasses by the rim or spoons by the bowl. They should never leave food exposed or sweet things open to flies.

Constant watchfulness, and teaching by example and patient repetition by those who understand the dangers of infected food or feeding utensils are essential. No nurse who has been taught *and has understood* should allow herself to become weary of the constant effort needed to secure a high standard of hygiene where service of food and drink is concerned.

11 MICROBIOLOGY APPLIED TO NURSING PROCEDURES

NURSING is carried out in certain definite units, not necessarily all of them in hospital, but whether the situation is the hospital ward, the home, the surgery, or the dispensary, the same basic principles will apply to all. Streptococci from a sore throat can be coughed into exposed milk in both the ward kitchen or the home kitchen; the effect is the same on those drinking it if they are susceptible to the organism and the dose. This is cross infection primarily of an airborne type, though in the infected person the bacteria may affect the gastro-intestinal tract. Unwashed hands may distribute this infection still further either after a ward sanitary round or a visit to the toilet in the ward or the home. The agents on this occasion are the faeces and the hands. Infected hands will carry infection to food in any kitchen, whether it is attached to a ward or to a dining room, and soiled hands are probably as often the vectors of pathogenic organisms as the readily blamed fly. Nevertheless, though many types of infection are common to a number of situations, many are of special importance to one department or another of the hospital service and a few of these special aspects of infection are the subject of this chapter.

Surgical and Medical Wards

There is no doubt that nurses whether trained or in training are familiar with the term 'cross infection'.

149

Ask a student nurse how cross infection is prevented and she will respond quite readily. She will say that prevention is achieved by the autoclaving of dressings, packs and other equipment, the wearing of masks, the washing of hands, and a strict non-touch technique both in setting the trolley and changing the dressings of patients. She will probably fail, to realize however, that the amount of space between beds is an important factor in the prevention of cross infection, she may not mention ventilation, she may not think of sore throats among the ward staff, she may not refer to the stye on a nurse's eye, a septic finger or an apron worn by a nurse among crowds in the street and then in the ward, as other possible sources of organisms.* As regards her hair, she may wilfully disregard the lesson she should have learnt when she saw all the organisms grown on the agar plate over which she shook her head. She may discuss the importance of dust thrown up by bedmaking or sweeping, and the timing of the ward dressing round after it, if there is no separate dressing room. However, she may not have grasped the relative importance of careful disinfection of bed linen subsequent to the discharge of a patient treated for, say, boils as compared with that of a non-infectious patient who has died of, say, heart failure, where conscientious social cleanliness is perfectly adequate.

To sum up, the practice of a safe aseptic technique is of the first importance, but its value can be seriously jeopardized by lack of understanding, integrity or ward discipline in any type of ward or situation, especially, it must be emphasized again, where there are sick or injured people.

There is another factor that is missed by people who

---

* Conversely nurses can carry pathogenic ward organisms on uniform or shoes (ward dust is heavily infected) into shops and public transport, etc. Mufti for shopping is a safe rule and protects the public.

think of infection as something that is always transmitted. This is not so, since bacteria are commonly found
in many parts of the body (see Chapter 8). For example,
the skin is the natural habitat of staphylococci, and
streptococci are found there too since some parts of the
body are perpetually exposed to the dust and bacteria-
laden atmosphere. Streptococci inhabit the throat, pneumococci the lungs and the *Escherichia coli* forms a normal
constituent of the faeces. The *Staphylococcus albus* is
harmless in the healthy conjunctival sac. The tissue
hosts and the parasitic organisms are, as it were, perfectly matched as long as the tissues are healthy, but this
equilibrium may easily be upset. Trauma of tissue, e.g.
scratching of the skin as a result of dirt or some other
irritant, poor aeration of the lungs due to faulty posture,
perhaps in bed, debility of tissue due to faulty circulation
of blood—any of these (and many other causes which
can easily be thought out) may reduce the natural
resistance of the host and give the organism the chance
for rapid development; hence the boil, the hypostatic
pneumonia, the bedsore. The good nurse who grasps
cause and effect can prevent many of these complications
occurring in her patients whatever may be the type of
illness or the difficulty of the situation. This is in no
sense a matter of cross infection, but it is quite as
important an aspect of the nurse's protective care of her
patient.

There is another problem which particularly affects
the patient in bed. Here again the nurse's understanding
of basic principles may be of the greatest service to her
patients. Bacteria will always multiply rapidly in waste
matter which is lying about in conditions favourable
to organic growth, that is where there is moisture and
warmth. The blood stream can carry bacteria to every
part of the body. Hence a haematoma under a surgical
wound, residual urine in a partially obstructed or

partially emptied bladder, excess fluid in a joint, are all liable to infection and a nurse must always be aware of this and be most careful in her observation and reporting on the condition of patients in whom these or other similar complications may occur. It is, of course, equally true that gross trauma of surface structures as in burns, scalds or crush wounds, by the destruction of tissue which occurs, also provides the ideal situation in which bacteria can flourish, and the most scrupulous asepsis must be observed.

The covering of the brain and spinal cord is a structure with poor resistance to infection and here again, in connection with intrathecal puncture and injections, the nurse's understanding and attention to detail is of paramount importance. Any lack of care in the cleansing of the patient's skin, the use of unsterile needles (for these procedures they should always be dry-sterilized or autoclaved) or any other failure in surgical technique may lead to most serious intrathecal infection.

From these observations it is clear that a patient may succumb in any ward to infection conveyed in two ways, i.e. by cross infection and/or auto-infection, and it is often practically impossible to determine which has occurred. Generally speaking any secondary infection of a clean wound is regarded as an example of cross infection and a condition which should not have occurred. Others, such as respiratory tract infections, are more difficult to assess unless there has been an obvious source of infection, such as a nurse, doctor, ancillary worker or visitor with a sore throat, cold or influenza.

Paediatric Wards

All that has been said about general wards applies to children's wards, with some important additions. Babies and young children have had less time than adults to develop immunity to infection and are therefore more susceptible to infection. For this reason they are best nursed at home. If, however, they have had to be admitted to hospital they must be rigorously guarded against cross infection. They must be nursed in glass walled cubicles; their nurses may be required to wear masks; and no one with a cold or a sore throat should be allowed near them.

Babies under one year are particularly prone to gastroenteritis because the acid defence of the hydrochloric acid in the gastric secretion is still lacking. It is therefore desirable that the nurses who change the babies' napkins should not prepare the feeds or the meals. If such an arrangement of staff duties is not feasible the most particular cleansing of the hands must be performed by the nurse after carrying out toilet duties and before proceeding to the kitchen or milk room. Obstinately retained long pointed nails may be especially serious in that they conserve virulent organisms and can readily damage a baby's delicate skin; they should never be tolerated in the nursery or kitchen of a paediatric ward. The danger of flies in the summer must not be forgotten either, and soiled napkins must be disposed of immediately in bin or antiseptic, and all milk feeds and food must be kept covered until the last moment. It is always desirable that milk feeds should be prepared in a special milk room and autoclaved and that specially prepared utensils, clean cloths and a washable table should be available for their preparation. The nurse is often gowned and masked. In the home less vigorous precautions are practised because a baby is on his own ground at home and is surrounded only by the organisms to which he is already used. This does not mean that scrupulous cleanliness is not necessary, and rapid disposal of soiled napkins and protection against flies is still important. The Milton technique of sterilization of feeding bottles is often used.

After having been washed and rinsed thoroughly, the bottles are completely submerged in a 1 in 80 solution of Milton antiseptic (electrolytic sodium hypochlorite solution), and left there until they are again required for use. The teats are also submerged in the Milton solution.

A further serious danger for young children is the occurrence of respiratory disease, since babies and very young children lack the strength to cough up sputum. This is another reason why no nurse, doctor or any other person with a sore throat or a cold should approach a baby without an effective mask.

Midwifery Ward

Whether a nurse is working in the midwifery department as a part of her experience during general training or whether she is taking her midwifery training, she should realize that here too there are some special aspects of infection.

The vulva of the patient during and after delivery must be kept scrupulously clean because the vagina which opens on to it leads up to the uterus where the separation of the placenta has left a large raw surface, very open to infection. In particular no nurse or doctor with a cold or sore throat should be allowed in the labour ward or with the newly delivered mother or baby. Haemolytic streptococci from the throat can produce puerperal fever in the newly delivered mother.

There is also the possibility of *Escherichia coli* from the rectum passing up the urethra and into the bladder if the area is not kept very clean. The skin around perineal stitches can also be infected if the area is allowed to become moist. It is therefore essential to keep the skin dry and clean to prevent breakdown of the wound.

Cracking of the nipples owing to lactation can result in a breast abscess as staphylococci may invade through the abrasion, and here again the nurse by vigilant super-vision and care can help in its prevention. It should be remembered in this connection that the umbilical stump of the baby is normally a healthy carrier site of staphy-lococci. Nipples that have been washed and carefully dried are less liable to crack and the nurse can provide for this precaution to be taken.

Many other examples of this kind of application of bacteriology to nursing will come to the mind of the thoughtful student, for example the care of the baby's eyes, scrupulous drying of his delicate skin particularly behind the ears and in the folds of the groins, the axillae and the buttocks, and the avoidance of thrush (*Candida albicans*) by ensuring that only clean objects go into his mouth.

In all these matters the nurse may be teaching, admon-ishing or merely setting an example, but one of her most potent weapons, for better or for worse, is the example she sets.

The Operating Theatre

The principles practised in the wards and other depart-ments of the hospital in preventing infection are equally applicable to the theatre, though here again there are some specific aspects which merit particular considera-tion. Wounds are made and sutured in the theatre, the débridement of bruised and lacerated tissue is carried out and internal organs are exposed and worked over for long periods of time. In none of these cases should it be possible for primary or secondary infection to occur. It is against these two possibilities with a full understanding of all the possible sources of infection, that the careful technique of the theatre is built up.

Thus the air in the theatre is usually filtered, warmed and moistened before entry and positive pressure

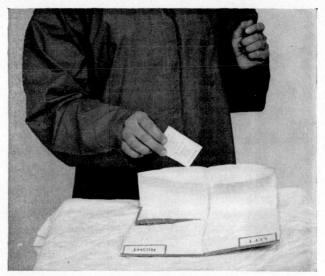

FIG. 44.—UNDO FIRST FOLDS OF GLOVE WRAPPER. TAKE POWDER ENVELOPE.

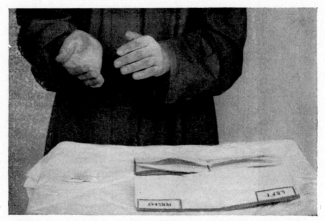

FIG. 45.—POWDER HANDS (POWDER MUST NOT FALL ON GLOVES).

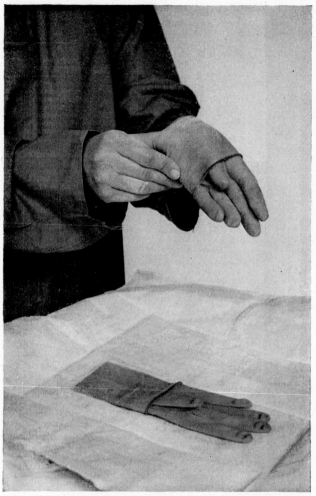

FIG. 46.—PICK UP LEFT GLOVE BY INSIDE OF WRIST. DRAW
ONTO HAND.

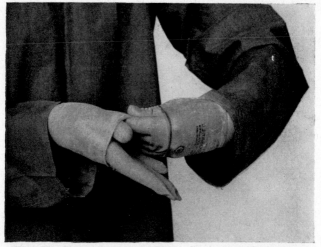

FIG. 47.—PLACE OUTSIDE OF FIRST GLOVE INTO OUTSIDE OF
SECOND AND DRAW IT ON TO THE HAND.

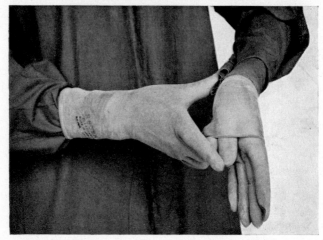

FIG. 48.—PLEAT OVER CUFF OF GOWN AND HOLD WITH
THUMB AS FINGERS PULL WRIST OF GLOVE OVER IT.

ventilation has been shown to achieve the best control of bacterial infection. The walls and floor of the theatre are washable, the juncture between wall and floor is curved and there is a wide gully with a slight slope to the outlet to take away all water used for washing floors between one case and the next or at the end of the list. Ideally, showers are provided for the use of all the theatre team. Staff entering the theatre prepared for an operating session wear special boots. In most theatres, because of the high temperature necessary to keep the exposed patient warm and partly in the interests of hygiene, the nurses and doctors discard outer clothing and wear special gowns only. All assisting with the operation wash hands and forearms thoroughly for three minutes and dry them on a clean towel before donning gowns, masks and sterile gloves The best method of putting on sterile gloves which prevents the skin of the hands from touching the outside of the gloves is shown in Figs. 44–48. Most surgeons either use Phisohex liquid for washing or apply Hibitane cream before putting on their gloves. Special caps are worn so that the hair of both doctors and nurses is completely covered. Dressings are autoclaved, instruments are autoclaved, boiled for five minutes or dry-sterilized in a hot air oven and syringes are autoclaved or dry-sterilized.

The patient's skin is prepared in the ward. This procedure involves at least a close shave and a bath, or a shave and a thorough cleansing with soap and water if the patient is not well enough to be bathed. The cleansing of the part of the body surface to be operated on, including the umbilicus, must be most carefully carried out since all adherent particles, bacteria, dead cells, sebum and sweat must be removed without damage to the skin. Some surgeons require no further preparation in the ward; others still prefer skin cleansing with a detergent antiseptic followed by spirit, or triple dye, iodine 2% in spirit, or some similar antiseptic painted on the skin and the whole area covered with a sterile towel and bandage. The argument for omitting the antiseptic is that these agents may irritate and dry the skin and are no more efficacious in removing bacteria than the thorough wash with soap and water. In either case an antiseptic is used to swab the skin in all operations immediately before the first incision is made.

The theatre list is always arranged so that clean types of operation, e.g. the clean stitch appendix, precede so called 'dirty' cases, e.g. colostomy, and the theatre is entirely washed down and everything washed and autoclaved if a spore bearing organism is introduced into the theatre, as might happen when a patient with gas gangrene is admitted for emergency surgery.

There is also a very careful record kept of all swabs used. The packets are always prepared with a definite number inside; the number of packets opened is marked up, and all swabs used are hung on a special rack and counted and a check is made before a wound which leads into any cavity, such as the abdomen or chest, is sewn up. A retained gauze or wool swab will cause serious infection if left inside the body.

To sum up: theatre technique is designed to reduce to the absolute minimum the possibility of cross infection. The patient is brought to the theatre in as good a condition as possible; the healthier the patient the higher his resistance to infection. There must be no dust and no dust traps in the theatre. Furniture and shelves must be washed down and never dusted. The air must be clean, and soiled articles removed as soon as possible. The theatre staff must be healthy; anyone with a cold or a sore throat should be excluded. Many epidemics of cross infection have been traced to the streptococcal sore throat of a member of the staff who mistakenly struggled on with his (or her) work when he should have been in bed and away from his fellow men. All equipment is clean or sterilized, the method of preparation depending on the composition or function of the equipment. Soiled shoes, exposed hair, long nails, exposed clothing are all sources of infection and should never be seen in a clean theatre. Sterile rubber gloves must be in perfect order and must be discarded at once even if only the most minute hole is suspected. The preparation of the patient depends on the type of operation, but in all patients the hair must be covered, the skin area must be clean, a clean gown and clean cotton socks or stockings must be put on, and usually special theatre trolley covers, mattresses and coverings are used in the theatre. All talking and movement should be cut to a minimum during an operation.

The impression is sometimes gained from nurses that surgical technique must be of a higher standard in the theatre than in the wards and departments. This is surely a misapprehension. The rules of surgical technique and all precautions against infection must be conscientiously applied everywhere. The theatre technique is more comprehensive and the emphasis is different mainly because the length of time taken and the amount of tissue exposed is usually so much greater in the theatre and the patient's resistance is lowered by the anaesthetic. Hence the theatre is, as it were, the home and centre of that tradition of careful excellence, from the booted and gowned surgeon and shiny instruments to the very wheels of the trolleys, which is designed for the better care of the patient. The same principles, however, must be applied everywhere.

Isolation

Full isolation is understood to mean the precautions necessary to prevent spread of infection by providing for the sick person a separate room away from the general wards of a hospital, with separate staff, or in an infectious diseases hospital.

Ward isolation indicates the separation of the patient from others in an individual side room or cubicle.

Bed isolation involves the barrier nursing of a patient in a ward pending the confirmation of a provisional diagnosis of an infectious disease, or while waiting for a bed in an isolation ward or hospital.

It is most important that nurses should fully understand and support the methods used to reduce the spread of infection. The following rules, based on the principles already discussed in this book, may provide a satisfactory code of practice.

1. Masks

Masks are worn for all nursing procedures for patients nursed in either ward or bed isolation in order to protect those attending the patient. They are worn by the nurse to protect the patient while she is attending to surgical dressings, spinal or thoracic punctures, obstetric deliveries and when looking after premature babies. One mask should be worn for attending to one patient only, or for a maximum period of 30 minutes, or 20 minutes if it is a disposable mask.

2. Gowns

Gowns must be worn for the same procedures as masks with the addition of maternity nurseries. The following rules must be observed;

  (a) In open wards the gowns are kept inside the screens on pegs beside the bed.
  (b) In cubicles or isolation rooms the gowns are kept in the rooms.

Only the contaminated outer surface of the gown should be handled when removing it, care being taken that the hands do not touch the inside. The inside is regarded as being clean and for hanging must be folded inwards. The word 'inside' may be marked in red on the inside of the collar band as a reminder of the importance of this point.

3. Hands

The hands are scrupulously washed with soap and running water, before donning the gown and after removal of it and before any other object is touched. Hands should be *washed thoroughly* before preparing or giving drinks, meals or infants' bottle feeds, and before examining a patient; also after attending to the patient, dealing with excreta, changing napkins, handling used crockery or soiled linen, cleaning or dusting the room or collecting specimens, and after examining a patient.

Many hospitals are now using a soap containing hexachlorophene in wards and departments because of its effectiveness against Gram positive cocci, and Phiso-hex cream in the theatres.

4. Screens

Screens are regarded as clean and must be handled only with clean hands. In bed isolation glass screens may be kept round the patient's bed, and when he is receiving attention ordinary screens are set up outside the glass ones.

If curtains are used round beds these should be touched only with clean hands.

5. Utensils

Utensils are treated according to their composition and use:

(*a*) All used crockery and cutlery are boiled in a special sterilizer in the kitchen or autoclaved, unless disposable utensils are supplied.

(*b*) Washing bowls are kept separate from others when bed isolation is being carried out, and in the room or cubicle for isolation patients, and must receive terminal disinfection.

(*c*) Bedpans and urinals are boiled in special sterilizer after use or are kept separate in all isolation techniques. When heat disinfection is not possible they should be placed in a disinfectant solution after sluicing, and then rinsed before use. One of the cresol disinfectants, such as Jeyes' Fluid, 1 in 80 or Printol 1 in 100, is suitable for this purpose.

(*d*) Disposable sputum containers are in general use today. These should be covered with sawdust and burned in a closed stove or furnace. Where they are not provided sputum can be emptied in the sluice, the sputum mugs mopped with disinfectant and boiled for 5 minutes. With tuberculous patients particular care should be taken. If special sterilizers are not provided, mugs and sputum may be placed in the steam disinfector and disinfected at 15 lb pressure for 20 minutes. Mugs can then be sluiced and washed without risk.

6. Disposal of Excreta

Stools, urine, discharges and vomit from infectious patients are mixed with Lysol or Jeyes' Fluid, 1 in 20 and left for 1 hour, or if the patient has poliomyelitis chloros 1 in 20, before disposal down the sluice.

Infected sputum should be poured into a receptacle containing Jeyes' Fluid 1 in 10, and left for not less than 2 hours before being sluiced away, if special sterilizers for mugs and sputum, or steam disinfectors, are not available. Alternatively destructible cartons may be dealt with as outlined above.

7. Infected Linen

The following rules apply to all isolation techniques:

(*a*) Unsoiled linen is sent in bags to the laundry for disinfection and laundering.

(*b*) Soiled linen is placed in dry pails with lids, which are brought to the bedside, and covered. Pails are taken to a tank containing one of the white fluid disinfectants, e.g. Lysol or White Cyllin, strength 1 in 160 (i.e. 6 g to 1 litre) or Printol 1 in 100, in which they are placed for 12 to 24 hours. Sometimes a tank on wheels is provided and this can be taken to the bedside. The tank is then transferred to the laundry intact; alternatively, Lysol 1 in 40 may be used for 2 hours' soaking, but this is more extravagant.

(*c*) Paper handkerchiefs which can be burnt are ideal and these, after use, should be placed in destructible paper bags and not under pillows or in pockets. If linen ones are used these should be kept in a bowl at the bedside, soaked in disinfectant (white fluid 1 in 80, or chloroxylenol 1 in 80) and sent to the laundry for boiling.

(*d*) Napkins should be discarded into a sanitary bin containing white disinfectant, strength 1 in 160, in the ward, and dealt with in the laundry.

(*e*) Face masks should be discarded into a bowl of chloroxylenol solution, strength 1 in 80, Printol strength 1 in 100, Milton strength 1 in 80, or a similar disinfectant, washed, boiled, ironed and autoclaved, or discarded and burnt if paper.

8. Bedding

The following rules should be observed for all infected bedding.

(*a*) Blankets, mattresses and pillows are sent in a special bag to the steam disinfector or autoclave after use. They are disinfected by steam at 109° C (228° F) with 5 lb pressure for 30 minutes, or if the new type of high vacuum high temperature autoclave is in use, for $3\frac{1}{2}$ minutes at 124° C (273° F). Blankets can also be sterilized in steam in the modern autoclave at subatmospheric pressure and 80° C (176° F) for $3\frac{1}{2}$ minutes. In addition a measured quantity of formaldehyde vapour is introduced into the autoclave if the infection is due to spore-bearing organisms.

(b) Mackintoshes or waterproof sheets if disposable waterproof material is not used, air rings and rubber mattresses are soaked in Lysol 1 in 20, Roccal 1 in 10, cetrimide 1 in 20 (5%) or Printol 1 in 100 for 2 hours, and are then scrubbed with soap and water and dried. Oxygen tents are treated in the same way, and are aired after drying.

With high vacuum, high temperature autoclaves rubber goods can be sterilized at the same pressures and temperatures as linen, dressings, instruments and utensils, and for the same length of time. This is because with the more complete evacuation of air, oxidation does not take place, this being the cause of damage to rubber in the older types of autoclave.

9. Books and Toys

Books and toys either should be cheap so that they may be destroyed after use, or they should be capable of being washed and disinfected. They should be tied to the bed or cot so that they do not fall on the floor which, as a rule, is grossly contaminated. Washable toys, belonging to the ward, are best for hospital use. Pencils and crayons should not be passed from child to child and should, therefore, be reserved for older children who can understand the order not to lend them to others.

10. Floors

Floors contaminated with infected material should be

disinfected with a white disinfectant, such as White Cyllin, strength 1 in 10, or Steroxol, which is non-slip, using a mop and pail.

11. Terminal Disinfection

The following rules are applied:

(*a*) Thermometers are placed in phenol 1 in 80, Roxenol or Roccal 1 in 40 or Printol 1 in 100 for 1 hour.

(*b*) Stethoscopes are mopped with phenol 1 in 20 or Roxenol or Roccal 1 in 10, and are then washed with soap and water.

(*c*) Lockers, bedsteads and other furniture are scrubbed with soap and water after first being mopped with phenol 1 in 20 or cetrimide 1 in 100, or Savlon 1 in 200. (Mopping is done only to remove extraneous debris; it does not disinfect. Scrubbing and washing with soap and water ensures thorough cleansing, which is the most important part of disinfection.)

(*d*) Disposable oxygen masks should be used wherever possible; if BLB masks are used, they are mopped with phenol 1 in 20 or Roxenol or Roccal 1 in 10, or Savlon 1 in 100, and are then washed with soap and water.

(*e*) The cubicles and contents are sometimes subjected to a special spraying process with formalin or other bactericide and left for 12 to 24 hours. If the room and its contents are dirty, they should be washed with cetrimide 1 in 20 solution.

The room should be well aired. Paint and waterproof surfaces of furniture should be washed down and other furniture well polished. Floors should be washed and if necessary lightly polished.

APPENDIX I SOME COMMON PATHOGENIC BACTERIA

Pathogenic organism	Characteristics of genus to which organism belongs	Clinical disease
Streptococcus pyogenes (group A streptococcus)	Spherical or ovoid cells in pairs or chains. Gram +. Growth on media slight. Changes blood-containing media. Mostly aerobes and facultative anaerobes	Scarlet fever
		Tonsillitis, sinusitis
		Otitis media
		Meningitis
		Pneumonia and complications
		Wound infections, cellulitis or erysipelas
		Puerperal fever
		(All these may lead to *septicaemia*)
Streptococcus pneumoniae, *Diplococcus pneumoniae* (pneumococcus)	As above	Pneumonia and its complications
		Sinusitis
		Otitis media
		Meningitis
		Conjunctivitis
		Peritonitis
		Septic arthritis, osteomyelitis

Route of entry	Route of exit	Length of infectivity	Usual source of infection
Any route. Usually respiratory	Secretions from site of lesions; generally respiratory	Until secretions negative to laboratory tests for organism	Human cases and carriers
Respiratory tract	Respiratory and nasal secretions	Until culture from secretions negative	
From respiratory tract via auditory tube	Aural, nasal and respiratory secretions		
From respiratory tract via middle ear or sinus; may be blood infection	No exit, unless infection has spread from throat or ear		
Respiratory tract	Sputum		
Locally	Pus from lesion		
Locally at placental site	Lochia		
Respiratory tract	Sputum	Organism present in normal secretions. Infection only with contributory factor, e.g. congestion, poor air entry or damaged mucosa	Human cases and carriers
Respiratory tract	Nasal secretions		
From respiratory tract via auditory tube	Aural and respiratory secretions		
From middle ear or sinus; may be from blood stream	No exit unless there is discharge from ear or respiratory tract		
Direct to conjunctiva	Conjunctival secretions	Until organism no longer present in secretions	
Via vagina (before puberty) or blood stream	No route of exit	Non-infectious	
Blood stream (Bacteraemia common during pneumonia)	No route of exit	Non-infectious	

SOME COMMON PATHOGENIC BACTERIA—*continued*

Pathogenic organism	Characteristics of genus to which organism belongs	Clinical disease
Faecal-type streptococci Aerobic type	As *Str. pyogenes,* but normally present in the gut	Urinary tract infections Secondary invader in wounds
Anaerobic type	As above; strictly anaerobic	Puerperal sepsis
Staphylococcus aureus (coagulase-positive) staphylococcus)	Spherical cells in clusters. Gram +. On agar, white, yellow or golden colonies grow. Variation in bio-chemical activity and pathogenicity	Localized skin infections, i.e. boils, carbuncles, whitlows, impetigo. Deeper local infections, abscesses Osteomyelitis Otitis media Pneumonia Gastroenteritis
Neisseria gonorrhoeae (gonococcus)	Cocci in pairs like kidney-beans. Gram −. Strict parasites, growing poorly on ordinary media; well if medium contains serum	Gonorrhoea (*Male:* urethritis, epi-didymitis, prostatitis) (*Female:* urethritis, cervicitis, vulvovagin-itis, salpingitis) Arthritis Ophthalmia neonatorum
Neisseria meningitidis (meningococcus)	As above	Meningitis (cerebro-spinal fever or spotted fever) Septicaemia, giving rise to rash, arthritis and ophthalmitis

Route of entry	Route of exit	Length of infectivity	Usual source of infection
Via urethra	Urine		From organisms in gut
Local	Pus from lesion		
Locally at placental site	Lochia		Danger always present because organism normally present in gut
Direct contact with infected material	Pus from lesions	Until lesion dry and culture from site negative	Human cases and carriers
From superficial lesion, infected injection needle or blood stream	None till abscess incised; then in discharge	Until discharge ceases	
Blood stream	No route till lesion discharges	While lesion discharges	
Respiratory tract via auditory tube	Discharge from ear	Until discharge gives negative cultures	
Respiratory tract	Sputum	Until sputum gives negative culture	
Infected food, particularly carbohydrates, e.g. custard, ice cream	Faeces and vomit	Remaining food dangerous, but faeces and vomit considered possibly infectious	Infected food
Direct spread during intercourse; rarely by cut or lip	From discharges	Until bacteriologically negative	Human cases and carriers
Blood stream; secondary to urethral lesion	No route of exit	Not infectious unless primary lesion is active	
Direct spread from maternal urethral or vaginal secretions	Conjunctival secretions	Until discharge bacteriologically negative	
Respiratory tract to meninges via lymphatics from sinus or blood stream	Nasal secretions	Until nasal discharge bacteriologically negative	Human cases and carriers
Blood stream	Skin lesions	Until rash has disappeared and secretions bacteriologically negative	

SOME COMMON PATHOGENIC BACTERIA—*continued*

Pathogenic organism	Characteristics of genus to which organism belongs	Clinical disease
Corynebacterium diphtheriae	Gram + rods, in palisades; staining irregularly, with swollen ends. Aerobic or facultative anaerobic. Some produce powerful exotoxin	Diphtheria Organism infects nasal cavity, pharynx, tonsils, larynx, trachea; rarely conjunctiva, wound or vagina: toxin absorbed from these sites cause of disease
Mycobacterium tuberculosis (tubercle bacillus)	Slender rods, Gram +, acid-fast; stain with difficulty. Grow slowly on media containing egg	Tuberculosis: (a) pulmonary (b) cervical glands (c) alimentary tract These primary infections by lymphatic or bloodstream may cause: Miliary tuberculosis Meningitis Bone and joint lesions Kidney lesions Testicular lesions Fallopian tube and uterine lesions
Mycobacterium leprae	As above	Leprosy (a) cutaneous (nodular) (b) neural (anaesthetic)
Bacillus anthracis	Large aerobic, spore-bearing organisms. Gram +. In chains of rods. Liquefy gelatin	Anthrax (a) cutaneous (b) pulmonary (Wool-sorters' disease) May lead to fatal septicaemia
Clostridium tetani	Anaerobic, spore-bearing rods; Gram +; in soil and intestinal tract of higher animals; may decompose protein and carbohydrate and produce toxin	Tetanus Symptoms due to powerful neurotoxin

Route of entry	Route of exit	Length of infectivity	Usual source of infection
Respiratory tract	Respiratory secretions	Until sites bacteriologically negative	Cases, convalescent cases and carriers (usually in nose or throat)
Local	From secretions		
Respiratory tract	Sputum	Until sputum bacteriologically negative	Open cases
Respiratory tract	Not infectious	Not infectious	Open cases or infected milk
Milk or swallowed sputum	Faeces	Until stool negative	Infected milk or swallowed sputum
⎫ ⎬ By the ⎭ circulation	Any open lesion Not infectious Not infectious Not infectious Urine Menstrual fluid	Until organisms absent Until organism absent Until organism absent	As above
Direct contact	Skin lesions	Until skin scrapings are negative	Contact with open case
Through skin or mucous membrane	No route unless cutaneous lesion positive		
Direct contact	Skin lesions	Until bacteriologically negative	Primarily affects animals through contact with infected hides, furs, etc.
Inhalation of infected material	Sputum		
Direct contact with infected material			Contamination with soil containing spores

SOME COMMON PATHOGENIC BACTERIA—*continued*

Pathogenic organism	Characteristics of genus to which organism belongs	Clinical disease
Clostridium perfringens (*Clostridium welchii*) and related	As for *Clostridium tetani*	Gas gangrene: symptoms due to toxaemia and may lead to septicaemia
Clostridium botulinum	As for *Clostridium tetani*	Botulinism, a pure toxaemia; infected food contains toxins that are absorbed from gut
Actinomyces israeli	Filamentous branching organism, with clubbed ends. Gram +. Pathogenic strain Anaerobic and non-acid-fast	Subacute or chronic granulomatous disease in man and animals; with suppuration and fistulae; usually cervico-facial, thoracic, or abdominal
Treponema pallidum	Thin, delicate spiral organism 4–14 μ in length by 0.2 μ Actively motile. No flagella	Syphilis (a) Congenital

(b) Primary syphilis (Chancre)

Secondary syphilis

Tertiary syphilis Gummata, Dementia paralytica, Meningo-vascular. Cardiovascular tabes |
| *Leptospira icterohaemor-rhagiae* | Spiral organism with fine close set curves; ends sharply curled; grown in enriched medium | Weil's disease |

Route of entry	Route of exit	Length of infectivity	Usual source of infection
Direct contact with infected material	Discharge from lesion		Contamination of deep wound with soil. Clostridia present in faeces of normal animals and man
Infected food	None: organism grows in food, not in intestine		Rare. Usual source home-canned vegetables or home-cured meat
Through the mouth. By aspiration. Direct extension from abdomen, by ingestion	Discharge from lesions		
Through placenta	Secretions of respiratory tract, if lesions in nose or lungs	Until secretions negative; but organism outside the body	Syphilitic mother
Direct contact	Discharge from chancre	While lesions persist	Direct contact during coitus
By blood stream from primary chancre	Discharge from surface lesions, i.e. ulcers in mouth		
By blood stream in secondary stage and develops later	Not infectious except that surface gummata may discharge spirochaetes	While gummata discharge	
By ingestion or by abrasions in skin or mucous membrane	Urine	While urine culture positive usually after 7 days	Rats spread organism and excrete it in urine. Contaminated water. Common in sewer workers

SOME COMMON PATHOGENIC BACTERIA—*continued*

Pathogenic organism	Characteristics of genus to which organism belongs	Clinical disease
Borrelia vincentii	Delicate spiral organism; 3–8 irregular spirals; anaerobic	Vincent's angina, with a a fusiform bacillus
Escherichia coli (*Bacterium coli*)	Gram— rods; normal in gut of man and animals; some pathogenic in gut; some non-pathogenic there but pathogenic elsewhere Aerobic and facultatively anaerobic; some strains motile	Low-grade infections; urinary tract infections. Peritonitis Secondary infection of wounds, burns, etc.
Salmonella typhi *Salmonella paratyphi*	Gram— rods; difficult to distinguish from *coli;* actively motile with flagella showing if suitably stained	Enteric fever (typhoid and paratyphoid)
Salmonella typhimurium	As above Some pathogens of animals	Gastroenteritis
Shigella sonnei	As above but non-motile	Bacillary dysentery
Proteus vulgaris	As above; present in normal gut	Low-grade infections; urinary tract infections
Pseudomonas aeruginosa, *Pseudomonas pyocyanea* (*Bacillus pyocyaneus*)	As above	Wound infections (Blue pus)

Route of entry	Route of exit	Length of infectivity	Usual source of infection
Respiratory tract	Respiratory secretions	While lesions persist	Human carriers or cases
From gut via urethra	Urine		Normal habitat of gut: outside causes lesions in other parts of body; by faecal contamination
From gut after perforation	No route		
Direct contact	Secretions of lesion		
Ingested material contaminated by excretions of case or carriers	All secretions during septicaemia for first 2 weeks; faeces, urine, rash	Until faeces and urine bacteriologically negative for 3 consecutive tests; relapses common from organisms in marrow, spleen, gall bladder or lymph glands	Human carriers or cases
Ingestion of infected food or water	Vomit and faeces	Until faeces bacteriologically negative	Human or animal cases or carriers, via food, e.g. milk, eggs shellfish, water
Ingestion of infected food or water	Faeces	Until faeces bacteriologically negative	Contaminated food or water by human cases or carriers
Via urethra from gut	Urine		Usually reflects faecal contamination
Direct contact	Discharge of lesion		Organism present widely in water, soil, sewage and gut

SOME COMMON PATHOGENIC BACTERIA—*continued*

Pathogenic organism	*Characteristics of genus to which organism belongs*	*Clinical disease*
Klebsiella pneumoniae	Gram— rod; present in normal respiratory tract and gut	Respiratory tract infections, e.g. pneumonia
Haemophilus influenzae	Pleomorphic rod. Gram—; may be capsulated. Easily killed. Difficult to grow. Associated with virus infections; not cause of influenza	Secondary respiratory tract infections; infects respiratory mucosa damaged by influenza virus
		Conjunctivitis
		Meningitis in children
		Septic arthritis
Haemophilus pertussis, Bordetella pertussis	As above, but less exacting to grow	Whooping cough
Haemophilus ducreyi	Very exacting in growth requirements	Soft chancre
Brucella abortus	Small cocco-bacillus; Gram—; aerobic; growth improved by carbon dioxide	Undulant fever
Brucella melitensis	As above	Malta fever

Route of entry	Route of exit	Length of infectivity	Usual source of infection
Via urethra from gut	Urine		Endogenous i.e. from organs of the individual
Direct contact	Secretions from lesions		
Normally present in respiratory tract; may become pathogenic	Nasal and bronchial secretions		
Respiratory tract; may be present in normal person	Respiratory secretions		Endogenous or contact with carrier
Direct contact	Conjunctival secretion		Contact with carrier
Respiratory tract via blood stream	No exit		Endogenous or contact with carrier
As above	No exit		
Respiratory tract	Respiratory secretions	Until secretions bacteriologically negative	Cases
Direct contact	Discharge from chancre	Until lesion healed	During intercourse
Ingestion or direct contact with excreta	Usually no exit; occasionally in urine	Not infectious	From drinking unpasteurized milk
Ingestion of goat's milk	Usually no exit	Not infectious	From infected goat's excreta, to goat's milk

APPENDIX II

THE PROTECTION OF THE NURSE

KING EDWARD'S Hospital Fund for London in their memorandum on the 'Supervision of Nurse's Health' says:

'Hospitals have great responsibility, and equally great opportunity, in relation to the care of their staff. Responsibility, because it is essential for the protection and well-being of the patients that those who tend them should not only be free from infection but should also be physically and mentally fit. Opportunity, because there is no more favourable ground for the practice of the hospitals' teaching and preventive function—a function that has too often been crowded out by the immediate claims of the acutely ill and the urgency of staff shortage. Hospitals should be centres of education in healthy living, and it would be their great loss, as well as that of the community, if their work came to be regarded as curative only.

'The "occupational hazards" (mainly infection and undue fatigue), of those who tend the sick lend themselves readily to preventive measures and control.'

It would probably be true to say that their recommendations include many that have been put into effect in large numbers of hospitals and already at the time of the report existed in some. They include:

The appointment of a physician to the nursing staff whose responsibilities should be preventive as well as curative. He should be a member of the consultant staff with direct access to the Management Committee. Nursing staff should have free access to him and be able to see him alone.

Medical examinations: before entry a detailed medical

history and report from the candidates' own doctor—
and a dental certificate should be obtained. *After entry*
examination by the physician to the nurses should be
carried out.

X-ray should be taken and repeated at the end of six
months and then yearly.

Weight should be recorded 6 monthly.

Remedial gymnastics with emphasis on posture, methods
of lifting and care of the feet should be taught.

Some of the other points worthy of note have been
covered in this book. Nurses with minor illnesses, i.e.
sore throats, septic fingers, etc., should be taken off
duty. They should receive medical care in a suitable
surgery or sick bay and should not be allowed on duty
until passed as recovered by the physician. There should
be a suitably qualified sister in charge of the nurses'
health which would be her major responsibility. Proper
convalescence should always be ensured. Sick leave
should not be taken as part of annual leave. Immunization against smallpox and diphtheria should be carried
out before entry to hospital. A Mantoux test should be
given, and the offer of BCG immunization made if the
result is negative. Proper provision for nursing tuberculosis patients should be made, and the nurses should be
carefully taught full precautions in order to protect
themselves and their patients. Open tuberculosis should
preferably be nursed in a special unit rather than in
general wards. Hours of duty, meals, recreation and
accommodation should all provide the environment
recognized as essential for health.

It has been suggested that each hospital should have a
health clinic for *all* members of its staff so that the
preventive aspect of its teaching may be clearly seen in
action. Apart from safeguarding the patients the loss of
working hours by staff might be considerably reduced,
more than offsetting the cost of this service.

APPENDIX III

VACCINATION AND IMMUNIZATION

THERE is a circular (H.M. (61) 96) on routine immuniza-
tion against infectious diseases issued by the Minister of
Health on the advice of his Standing Medical Advisory
Council.

The diseases against which immunization is advised are
diphtheria, pertussis (whooping cough), tetanus, smallpox and poliomyelitis.

First it is pointed out in this paper that the human
infant cannot at birth produce antibodies in response to
antigenic stimulation and is unlikely to be able to do so
until six to nine months of age. A high level of maternally
transmitted antibody may also adversely affect the baby's
ability to form antibodies. Other practical points discussed aim at showing the best timing of vaccination as
regards safety, effectiveness and economy of time.

Mothers are more likely to respond, it is said, to
suggestions about immunization during the first months
of an infant's life. It is important for the sake of parents
and the domiciliary services that the number of visits
should be cut to the minimum that will give satisfactory
protection. In general the time when protection is needed,
judged by notification of infectious disease figures, is
between one and four years of age.

Resulting from these and other considerations a combined antigen consisting of diphtheria toxoid, tetanus
toxoid and pertussis vaccine, carefully balanced so that
each can produce a good antibody response may be
administered.

As from 1965, simultaneous poliomyelitis immunization with Sabin oral vaccine has been permitted with the triple vaccine (diphtheria-tetanus-pertussis).

Usual Scheme of Immunization

2–5 months old	3 doses of triple vaccine (DPT) and oral Sabin poliomyelitis at 4–6 week intervals
18–21 months	Booster dose of the above
12–24 months	Smallpox vaccination (with an interval of at least 3 weeks between it and any other immunization)
5 yrs (school entry)	Booster dose of diphtheria, tetanus and poliomyelitis immunization. (NOT pertussis)
8–12 yrs	Booster Diph-Tet, and re-vaccination
12 yrs or over	BCG

Reference: *On the State of the Public Health*, 1965.

COMMON TERMS
IN MICROBIOLOGY

EVERY student nurse should make a simple glossary in order to familiarize herself with difficult words. The best way to do this is to list every unknown term as it is discovered and either look it up in the dictionary or in some other way find out its meaning. This may have to be repeated several times before complete mastery is achieved. Then one could ask someone else to explain the word, thus testing one's own knowledge at the same time as ensuring theirs, a very good method of learning.

To show the kind of definition that might be included in the glossary, a few of the more difficult terms to be found in this book are defined below:

Anaerobe. A microorganism which can live without air or free oxygen.

Facultative anaerobe. A microorganism which can adopt itself to grow in presence of free oxygen but which does not grow as well as in anaerobic conditions.

Obligative anaerobe. A microorganism which can *only* live and grow in the absence of free oxygen.

Antibiotic. A chemical substance derived from living cells producing a bactericidal effect on other living cells.

Bacteriophage. A virus which attacks bacteria, one virus to one variety of bacterium. New viruses develop inside the specific bacterium which has been attacked and then burst out; each of the freshly released viruses then attacks a new bacterium.

Chemotherapy. Treatment using chemical substances

which affect pathogenic organisms without injuring body cells.

Coagulase.   The enzyme produced by a potentially pathogenic staphylococcus which coagulates human plasma.   The *Staphylococcus aureus* is said to be 'coagulase positive' because it produces this enzyme.   Other types of staphylococci are 'coagulase negative'.

Commensalism.   A situation in which two organisms live together to the benefit of one, the other not being affected.

Myxovirus.   A virus which has an enzyme capable of breaking down muco-protein.

Pleomorphic.   Occurring in many distinct forms.

Radical.   An atom or group of atoms able to combine as one unit with other atoms or groups.

Specific.   Pertaining to a particular species or disease.

Carrying on from these definitions it is suggested that those who have read this book carefully should be able to explain the meanings of the following words:

Agglutination	Immunity
Antibody	Incubation
Antigen	Infection
Antiseptic	Inorganic
Arbovirus	Organic
Aseptic	Parasite
Barrier nursing	Pathogen
Bed isolation	Plasma
Carrier	Saprophyte
Disinfection	Serum
Endotoxin	Sterilization
Exotoxin	Vaccine

This list is not meant to be exhaustive, but in making certain of the meanings of these terms old knowledge will be consolidated and new knowledge gained.

SELECTED FURTHER READING

Books

Baldry, P. E. (1965) *The Battle against Bacteria. A History of the Development of Antibacterial Drugs for the General Reader*. Cambridge University Press.

Bisset, K. A. (1963) *Bacteria*. 3rd ed. E. & S. Livingstone.

Brooks, S. M. (1962) *Basic Facts of Medical Microbiology*. 2nd ed. Saunders.

Cuny, H. (1965) *Louis Pasteur: The Man and His Theories*. Translated by Patrick Evans. Souvenir Press.

Drew, John (1940) *Man, Microbe and Malady*. Penguin.

Fairbrother, R. W. (1962) *A Textbook of Bacteriology*. 9th ed. Heinemann Medical Books.

Frobisher, M. and others (1964) *Microbiology for Nurses*. 11th ed. Saunders.

Gale, A. H. (1959) *Epidemic Diseases*. Penguin.

Garb, S. and Sporne, P. (1962) *Nurses' Manual of Laboratory Tests*. 1st English ed. Heinemann Medical Books.

Gillies, R. R. and Dodds, T. C. (1965) *Bacteriology Illustrated*. E. & S. Livingstone.

Guthrie, Douglas (1949) *Lord Lister. His Life and Doctrine*. E. & S. Livingstone.

Hare, Ronald (1967) *Bacteriology and Immunity for Nurses*. 2nd ed. Longmans, Green.

Hare, Ronald (1967) *An Outline of Bacteriology and Immunity*. 2nd ed. Longmans, Green.

Hynes, M. (1964) *Whitby and Hynes's Medical Bacteriology Including Elementary Mycology and Parasitology*. 8th ed. Churchill.

Manson-Bahr, Sir Philip (1962) *Patrick Manson—the Father of Tropical Medicine*. Nelson.

Marshall, Stanley (1965) *Elementary Bacteriology and Immunity for Nurses*. 4th ed. H. K. Lewis.

Parish, H. J. (1965) *A History of Immunization*. E. &. S. Livingstone.

Pinniger, J. L. and Tighe, J. R. (1967) *Pathology*. 2nd ed. Baillière, Tindall and Cassell.

Rowland, John (1953) *The Mosquito Man. The story of Sir Ronald Ross*. Lutterworth Press.

Rowland, John (1958) *The Microscope Man*. Lutterworth Press.

Smith, K. M. (1965) *The Biology of Viruses*. Oxford University Press.

Stewart, F. S. (1968) *Bacteriology and Immunology for Students of Medicine* (formerly Bigger's handbook of bacteriology). 9th ed. Baillière, Tindall and Cassell.

Taylor, I. and Knoweldon, J. (1964) *Principles of Epidemiology*. 2nd ed. Churchill.

Taylor, G. (1964) *Bacteriology for Nurses*. Heinemann Medical Books.

Thomas, C. G. A. (1968) *Medical Microbiology*. 2nd ed. Baillière, Tindall and Cassell.

Turk, D. C. and Porter, I. A. (1965) *A Short Textbook of Microbiology*. The English Universities Press.

White, R. G. (1963) *Essentials of Bacteriology*. Pitman Medical.

Whittet, T. D. and others (1965) *Sterilization and Disinfection*. Heinemann Medical Books.

Williams R. E. O. and others (1966) *Hospital Infection: Causes and Prevention*. 2nd ed. Lloyd-Luke.

Reports

Control of infections in hospitals: American Hospital Association Monograph Series No. 12, 1963.

Great Britain War Office—Memoranda on medical diseases in tropical and sub-tropical areas. H.M.S.O. Published in the 1940s. No up-to-date edition.

Control of communicable diseases in man. Official Report of the American Public Health Association. 10th ed. rev. by John E. Gordon, 1965.

Staphylococcal infections in hospital (1959) Ministry of Health report.

World Health Organization Reports

Food hygiene. Fourth Report of the Expert Committee on Environmental Sanitation. Technical Reports Series No. 104. 1956.

Joint FAO/WHO Expert Committee on Milk Hygiene. First Report. 1956. Technical Report Series No. 124. 1957.

Air Pollution. Fifth Report of the Expert Committee on Environmental Sanitation. Technical Report Series No. 157. 1958.

The role of immunization in communicable disease control. Public Health Papers No. 8. 1961.

Gonorrhoea. *WHO Bulletin*, vol. 24, No. 3, 1961.

Measles vaccines. Report of a WHO Scientific Group. Technical Report Series No. 263, 1963.

Smallpox. First report of an Expert Committee, 1964.

Nursing Times and Nursing Mirror articles

Ridley, M. 'Barrier nursing.' *N.T.* 16.3.62.

Broome, W. E. 'Isolation techniques.' *N.T.* 10.5.63.

Schwarz, Kurt 'Immunization 1964.' *N.T.* 9.10.64.

Levin, S. 'Bacteriology in the Bible.' *N.M.* 8.1.65.

Hughes, T. A. 'Planning and equipping a CSSD for a new hospital.' *N.T.* 19.3.65.

Carter, E. 'Automation in a CSSD.' *N.T.* 7.5.65.

Parry, Wilfred H. 'Diseases transmitted by pets.' *N.T.* 18.6.65.

'Immunology now—an explanation.' *N.T.* 3.9.65.

Parry, Wilfrid H. 'Hospital infection.' *N.T.* 24.9.65.

Gibson, M. and Mann, T. P. 'Barrier nursing for sick children. *N.T.* 24.9 and 1.10.65.

Lowbury, E. J. L. 'Research on control of hospital infection by air-conditioned isolation wards.' *N.T.* 12.11.65.

Winner, H. I. 'An introduction to microbiology.' *N.T.* 2.10, 9.10, 16.10, 23.10, 30.10.64.

Hare, Ronald 'Bacteriological methods in the diagnosis of various diseases.' *N.T.* 18.2.66.

Flewitt, T. H. 'Laboratory diagnosis of virus disease'. *N.T.* 25.3.66.

Winner, H. I. 'A bacteriologist looks at hospital bedding.' *N.T.* 22.4.66.

Sheahan, John 'Methods of sterilization and disinfection: a survey of current practice in 50 hospitals in England and Wales.' *N.T.* 17.6.66.

Parry, Wilfrid H. 'Milk-borne diseases.' *N.T.* 23.12.66.

Reading, B., and Brigden, R. J. 'A record system for CSSD.' *N.T.* 24.2.67.

Bradbeer, T. L., and others. 'The Infection Control Sister.' *N.T.* 26.5.67.

Donovan, J. 'Reverse barrier nursing: Care of patients with bone marrow depletion.' *N.T.* 16.6.67.

Parry, Wilfrid H. 'Hospital infection.' *N.T.* 24.9.67.

Index

INDEX

193

NURSING BOOKS

New Books

Bull & Isaacs

Do-it-Yourself Revision for Nurses: Books I and II

Do It Yourself Revision is an entirely new concept which provides the student nurse with a systematic and interesting method of revision by which she can study a particular subject, answer questions selected from recent State Final Examinations, and mark her replies against model answers provided.

Book 1   144 pages   4 illus.   10s.
Book 2   144 pages   7 illus.   10s.

Chisholm

An Insight into Health Visiting

This book by an experienced health visitor describes the daily routine of health visiting and how the often simple procedures she may carry out in the home are only the starting point of her real work as a health educator.

approx. 118 pages   approx. 18s.

Delilios et al.

Baillière's Handbook of First Aid

The sixth edition of this famous Handbook has been extensively revised by STANLEY MILES. While the comprehensive practical first aid instruction of the original authors, which has given the Handbook its reputation as a complete and authoritative work, has been retained, there has been considerable rewriting of the text to include the technical advances in cardiac and respiratory resuscitation and the treatment of shock and burns which have taken place recently.

6th edn.   approx. 400 pages   180 illus.   25s.

Mountjoy & Wythe

Nursing Care of the Unconscious Patient

This new book has been written to help nurses and others responsible for the care of patients whose level of consciousness is abnormal, for whatever reason and wherever the patient is being nursed.

illus.   104 pages   15s.

BAILLIÈRE, TINDALL & CASSELL LTD.

Reference Books

Baillière's
Nurses' Dictionary
By **BARBARA F. CAPE, S.R.N., S.C.M., D.Ñ.**

The latest edition of this ever-popular dictionary contains over 750 new definitions, and the 24 appendices are full of new information relating particularly to those subjects in which important developments are taking place.

17th Edition   572 pages   174 illustrations   10s.

Baillière's
Midwives' Dictionary
By **VERA DA CRUZ, S.R.N., S.C.M., M.T.D.**

This pocket dictionary, which has again been revised and brought up-to-date, is suitable both for midwives and for nurses taking their obstetric option. Obsolete terms have been omitted to provide space for new data, and the appendices have been heavily revised or rewritten.

Baillière's
Pocket Book of Ward Information
By **MARJORIE HOUGHTON, O.B.E., S.R.N., S.C.M., D.N.**

Fully revised and brought up-to-date, this book contains a multitude of useful information likely to be needed by nurses in their day to day work and of particular help to nurses in training.

9s.

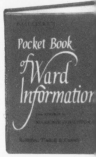

BAILLIÈRE, TINDALL & CASSELL, LTD

CONCISE MEDICAL TEXTBOOKS

modern series of inexpensive and authoritative textbooks
ritten primarily for medical students, which will provide the
ained nurse with sound and accurate knowledge of the special-
ed branches of medicine in which she may be interested.

NDERSON & TRETHOWAN
PSYCHIATRY
E. W. ANDERSON, M.D., M.SC.,
R.C.P., D.P.M., and W. H.
ETHOWAN, M.B., F.R.C.P.
OND), F.R.A.C.P., F.A.N.Z.C.P.,
P.M.
d ed.   328 pages   28s.

RAIGMYLE
EMBRYOLOGY
M. B. L. CRAIGMYLE, M.B.,
.B., M.D.
illus.   216 pages   25s.

ATTA & OTTAWAY
IOCHEMISTRY
S. P. DATTA, B.SC., M.B., B.S., and
H. OTTAWAY, B.SC., PH.D.,
R.I.C.
d ed.   77 illus.   378 pages   30s.

OLMES
OBSTETRICS
d ed.   37 illus.   256 pages   28s.
d

GYNAECOLOGY
J. M. HOLMES, M.D., B.S. (LOND),
R.C.O.G.
illus.   236 pages   25s.

AW
RGANIC CHEMISTRY
G. A. MAW, D.SC., PH.D., F.R.I.C.
4 pages   25s.

ULIAN
CARDIOLOGY
D. G. JULIAN, M.A., M.D.,
R.C.P.E., M.R.C.P., M.R.A.C.P.
5 illus.   365 pages   35s.

MACKENNA & COHEN
DERMATOLOGY
By R. M. B. MACKENNA, M.A., M.D.,
B.CHIR. (CANTAB.), F.R.C.P., and
E. LIPMAN COHEN, M.A., M.B.,
B.CHIR.
1 plate   288 pages   28s.

MEREDITH DAVIES
**PUBLIC HEALTH AND
PREVENTIVE MEDICINE**
By J. B. MEREDITH DAVIES, M.D.,
D.P.H.
5 illus.   26 tables   318 pages   30s.

PINNIGER & TIGHE
PATHOLOGY
By the late J. L. PINNIGER, revised by
J. R. TIGHE, M.D., B.SC., M.R.C.P.,
M.R.C.P.E., M.C.PATH.
2nd ed.   288 pages   28s.

THOMAS
MEDICAL MICROBIOLOGY
By C. G. A. THOMAS, M.A., B.M.,
B.CH.(OXON.), M.R.C.P., M.C.PATH.
2nd ed.   388 pages   28s.

WYBAR
OPHTHALMOLOGY
By KENNETH WYBAR, M.D., CH.M.,
D.O.M.S., F.R.C.S.
79 illus.   360 pages   30s.

PENN
PHARMACOLOGY
By R. G. PENN, M.B., B.CH. (WALES).
14 illus.   300 pages   30s.

& 8 Henrietta Street, London WC2.

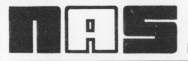 **NURSES' AID SERIES**

ANATOMY AND PHYSIOLOGY FOR NURSES
by Katharine E. Armstrong, S.R.N., S.C.M., D.N.

7th edn.   14s.

ANAESTHETICS FOR NURSE
by Joan Hobkirk, S.R.N.

1st edn.   *in preparatio*

ARITHMETIC IN NURSING
by Wm. C. Fream, S.R.N., B.T.A., CERT.

3rd edn.   15s.

EAR, NOSE AND THROAT NURSING
by S. Marshall, S.R.N., S.C.M., D.N.

4th edn.   16s

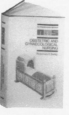

New Edition

OBSTETRIC AND GYNAECOLOGICAL NURSING
by R. E. Bailey, S.R.N., S.C.M., M.T.D., R.N.T., D.N.

1st edn   hard cover 20s
                   paperback 14

MEDICAL NURSING
by Marjorie Houghton, O.B.E., S.R.N., S.C.M., D.N., and Mary Whittow, S.R.N.

7th edn.   hard covers 24s.
                paperback 16s.

MICROBIOLOGY FOR NURSE
by E. J. Bocock, S.R.N., S.C.M., D.N. R.T.N., and K. F. Armstrong, S.R.N., S.C.M., D.N.

3rd edn.   16s

PAEDIATRIC NURSING
by M. A. Duncombe, S.R.N., R.S.C.N, S.C.M., and B. Weller, S.R.N., R.S.C.N., R.N.T.

3rd edn.   hard cover 24s
                paperback 16

ORTHOPAEDICS FOR NURSES
by W. Talog Davies, S.R.N., S.C.M.

3rd edn.   16s.

BAILLIÈRE, TINDALL & CASSELL, LTD

…series of complete illustrated textbooks covering the requirements of the …C. Examination syllabus, each volume being written by an expert on the …ject. New volumes or editions may have been added; up-to-date information … gladly be supplied on request.

…ACTICAL PROCEDURES

…. Houghton, O.B.E., S.R.N.,
…M., D.N., and J. E. Parnell, S.R.N.,
…M., R.N.T.

…edn.   *12s.*

PHARMACOLOGY FOR NURSES
by Rosemary E. Bailey, S.R.N.,
S.T.D., D.N.

2nd edn.   *16s.*

…ACTICAL NURSING

…arjorie Houghton, O.B.E., S.R.N.,
…M., D.N., and Mary Whittow,
…N.

… edn.   *14s.*

PSYCHOLOGY FOR NURSES
by A. Altschul, B.A., S.R.N., R.M.N.

3rd edn.   *hard cover 20s.*
                     paperback 14s.

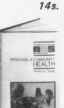

…d Edition

PERSONAL AND COMMUNITY HEALTH
by Winifred L. Huntly, S.R.N., S.C.M.,
D.N.

2nd edn.   *hard cover 16s.*
                     paperback 10s.

…CHIATRIC NURSING

…. Altschul, B.A., S.R.N., R.M.N.

…edn.   *hard cover 24s.*
                     paperback 16s.

SURGICAL NURSING
by Katharine F. Armstrong, S.R.N.,
S.C.M., D.N., and Norna Jamieson,
M.A., S.R.N., S.C.M., S.T.D., revised
by Peggy Sporne, S.R.N., D.N., R.N.T.

8th edn.   *hard cover 24s.*
                     paperback 16s.

…EATRE TECHNIQUE

…arjorie Houghton, O.B.E., S.R.N.,
…M., D.N., and Jean Hudd, S.R.N.

…edn.   *16s.*

TROPICAL HYGIENE
by Wm. C. Fream, S.R.N., B.T.A.
CERT., S.T.D.

5th edn.   *16s.*

& 8 Henrietta Street, London WC2.

Standard Textbooks

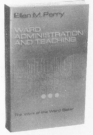

WARD ADMINISTRATION & TEACHIN[G]
By Ellen L. Perry

"This is a book which has long been needed. Every trai[n]
nurse could learn something from it. While ward sisters [put]
into practice the ideals and ideas outlined, we need have [no]
fears for 'patient care' in our hospitals nor for the pract[ical]
training of the nurse."   *Nursing Mir[ror]*

304 pages   *11 illus.*   3[...]

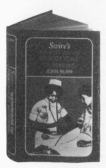

SWIRE'S HANDBOOK
OF PRACTICAL NURSING
Revised by Joan Burr

Changes in the syllabus of training have necessitate[d a]
major revision for this edition and Miss Burr has taken [the]
opportunity to make many changes of approach to st[ress]
the human angle and to enable the nurse to appreciate [her]
surroundings in the hospital and in the community. C[are]
has been taken to cover the syllabus fully, and the use [of]
simple language and illustrated example ensures [the]
maintained interest of the pupil.
6th Edition

308 pages   *57 illus.*   2[...]

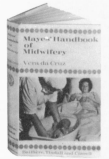

MAYES' HANDBOOK
OF MIDWIFERY
Revised by V. Da Cruz

"In this Seventh Edition, Miss da Cruz has incorpora[ted]
the many new trends and advances made in recent years[...]
The text is set out with clear headings and good illustrati[ons]
which make revision easy."   *Maternal and Child C[are]*

458 pages   3[...]
156 illus.   *10 pla[tes]*

BAILLIÈRE, TINDALL & CASSELL, LT[D]

library of textbooks specially written for the trained nurse studying for specialist qualifications and for the young nurse who is just beginning her training.

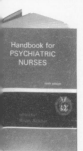

HANDBOOK FOR PSYCHIATRIC NURSES
Edited by the late Brian Ackner

"The R.M.P.A. is to be congratulated on sustaining its great tradition in nursing education by re-modelling its famous 'Handbook' to produce an entirely new account of psychiatry for nurses . . . this is an extremely readable and useful book."
9th Edition   *Nursing Mirror*

364 pages   *1 illus.*   *35s.*

NURSING THE PSYCHIATRIC PATIENT
By Joan Burr

"This book has rapidly been acclaimed as an excellent addition to the psychiatric nursing textbooks already available, and it certainly provides a masterly account of what caring for the mentally ill is about. . . . it is written with such sympathy that, should somebody recognise a description of their own difficulties, they could well gain comfort from the fact that such a helpful understanding is being disseminated."   *Nursing Times*

                                                    cased 25s.
308 pages   *10 illus.*   *paperback 16s.*

BERKELEY'S PICTORIAL MIDWIFERY
Revised by D. M. Stern

A pictorial survey with excellent illustrations accompanied by clear descriptive text, which will prove invaluable to both the student and qualified midwife alike.

The book has a dual role, providing a text and atlas of theory and a reference for the practical aspects of the subject.
". . . a standard book which every nursery and, if possible, every student nursery nurse should possess . . .".
                                                    The Medical Officer

176 pages   *25s.*
224 illus.   *2 coloured plates*

& 8 Henrietta Street, London WC2.

BAILLIÈRES
Anatomical Atlases

By Katharine Armstrong, S.R.N., S.C.M., D.N., and Douglas J. Kidd, M.M.A.A.

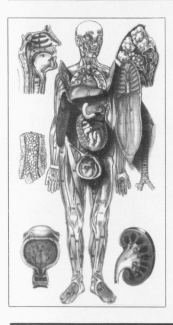

Atlas of Female Anatomy

7th Edition

In the illustration shown here, stick-on flaps showing the abdominal organs can be affixed which lift up to reveal the parts beneath. Each internal organ is thus fully visible and its exact relationship to other organs is clear. Although Miss Armstrong's terminology and presentation remain virtually the same, the publishers have taken the opportunity, with the publication of the 7th edition, of revising the text and index where modern practice and usage have seemed to make it necessary. The introductory text has been revised to allow the reader a page size of greater convenience and ease of study. The colour plates remain unchanged.

25s.

Atlas of Male Anatomy

5th Edition

The Male Atlas retains its original format ; printed in full colour, it shows clearly the full size, shape, position and detail of every part and structure of the human body. Great attention has been paid to accuracy of detail even in the smallest illustrations, with a key index naming every part and a clear and concise explanatory text.

25s.

Baillière's Atlases provide the geography of the human body at a glance and learning easy ; they are indispensable to all nurses as a means of simple and sp reference.

(Postage 2s. 6d. e

BAILLIÈRE, TINDALL & CASSELL LT